CW01496655

The 1836 London Diary Of James Stratton Carpenter MD

Edited and Annotated by

T REED FERGUSON

MINERVA PRESS
WASHINGTON   LONDON   MONTREUX

THE 1836 LONDON DIARY OF JAMES STRATTON
CARPENTER MD
Copyright © T Reed Ferguson 1996

ISBN 1 86106 230 3

First Published 1996 by
MINERVA PRESS
195 Knightsbridge
London SW7 1RE

Printed in Great Britain by
B.W.D. Ltd., Northolt, Middlesex

The 1836 London Diary Of
James Stratton Carpenter MD

T Reed Ferguson, retired Vice President of the Pennsylvania State University, married Cornelia Stratton Carpenter, the great great granddaughter of Dr James Stratton Carpenter during the early days of World War II. He was teaching Art History, Drawing and Painting at a branch of the University at Pottsville, Pennsylvania where the author of the diary started practising medicine in 1830. Dr Carpenter was succeeded by three generations of physicians in the same town (1830-1969) including Mrs Ferguson's father.

Reed Ferguson served with the American Red Cross at Pearl Harbor, Hawaii during the latter days of the war and returned to Pottsville after the armistice. Shortly thereafter, the university asked the Fergusons to start a new campus in Erie, Pennsylvania, now a four year college.

Returning to the main campus of the university in 1954, Reed Ferguson became involved in administration, ending his career as Vice President for Public Affairs in 1975. The Fergusons spent the next eighteen years travelling the world, serving as volunteers in local hospitals, local museums and historical societies. Mr Ferguson researched and wrote a historical biography which was published by Mercer University Press, *The John Couper Family At Cannon's Point*.

A year or so before Mrs Ferguson passed away (August 1992), she found the James Stratton Carpenter's London diary among some family books. Reading the diary, using a magnifying lens lamp, her husband put it on the computer. After Cornelia's death, he started editing the diary, carrying on extensive research by letter and telephone, finally spending several weeks in London. He visited the same locations as Dr Carpenter had: hospitals and medical schools where he had attended lectures, theatres, restaurants (none of which exist today), and the historic monuments such as Hampton Court Palace, Westminster Abbey, St Paul's Cathedral, Greenwich, the Houses of Parliament, and the bridges of London.

The diary is documented in the Fergusons' files with a copy of Dr Carpenter's medical school thesis, a copy of the French Patent he secured for the belt to cure Hernia, copies of four London newspapers carrying his advertisement as well as many letters identifying the source of material.

Introduction

James Stratton Carpenter was a great, great grandson of the first Carpenter to come to the United States from England, a man named Samuel Carpenter.

It is not clear where Samuel and his brothers Joshua and Abraham came from, but it seems likely that it was from the Sussex area. However, they were apparently men of some means and education, which was remarkable for the early seventeenth century. Samuel had succeeded in the sugar industry in Barbados for ten years before going to the Quaker Pennsylvania Colony. He had joined the Quaker Society before leaving England, although his two brothers remained members of the Church of England.

The Charter of Pennsylvania was granted by Charles II to William Penn on January 5th 1681. The first emigrant ship, *The John and Sarah*, arrived in Delaware in the autumn of 1681, and the city of Philadelphia was established in the latter part of 1682.

William Penn arrived at New Castle on 27th October 1682, and in the same year, twenty-three ship loads of emigrants and supplies arrived in Delaware.

Samuel Carpenter arrived in July 1683. Among the records in the Race Street Friends Meeting House of Philadelphia, is a certificate of acceptance of Samuel Carpenter from the 'Friends at Bridgetown in the Island of Barbados, the 23rd day of the 6th month 1683'. The original of the marriage certificate of Samuel Carpenter and Hannah Hardiman, written on parchment and dated December 12, 1684, is preserved in the Historical Society of Pennsylvania.

The name of Samuel Carpenter appears prominently in the early history of Philadelphia and Pennsylvania; he is listed as treasurer of the Province of Pennsylvania. He is mentioned in Proud's *History of Pennsylvania*.

Samuel Carpenter arrived early in Pennsylvania and was one of the most considerable traders and settlers. He held for many years some of the greatest offices of the Government, and through a great variety of business he preserved the love and esteem of a large number of acquaintances. His great abilities, activity and benevolent disposition of mind in divers capacity, but more particularly among his friends the Quakers, are said to have rendered him a very useful member not only of the religious society, but of the community in general.

A letter written by Samuel Carpenter to William Penn in 1702 is addressed, 'Dear Friend and Governor William Penn' and signed, 'Thy real friend.' William Penn is known to have stayed with the Carpenters for a month or so during his second trip to Philadelphia. They lived in a house known as the 'Slate Roof House'.

All of the early Carpenters who succeeded Samuel were prominent in government and industry in and around Philadelphia. These include Samuel Carpenter II, Preston Carpenter, and Thomas Carpenter. Thomas was active in the Revolutionary War with service in General Washington's Army in 1777. Following the war, he established a Glass Manufacturing business carried on by his son, Edward Carpenter, in Glassborough, New Jersey.

Edward Carpenter married Sarah Stratton in 1799, daughter of Dr James Stratton, and these were the parents of James Stratton Carpenter, born on October 18th 1807.

There is little information concerning James Stratton Carpenter, except that he studied medicine with a Dr Joseph Fithian of Woodbury New Jersey and then graduated from the University of Pennsylvania Medical School in 1829 with an MD. His thesis on file in the medical school library, was on Acute Hepatitis. He immediately started a lucrative medical practice in Pottsville, Schuylkill County, Pennsylvania, and married Camilla Julia Sanderson October 12th 1832.

Camilla's father was John Sanderson, who was born near Carlisle, Cumberland County, Pennsylvania. He was educated by private tutors and studied law, but he finally devoted himself to literature, and became an associate instructor in the Clermont Seminary, where the principal was John Thomas Caree. Sanderson married Caree's daughter, Sophie, and they had ten children. Due to poor health, John Sanderson went abroad in 1835 and when he returned he was made professor of Latin and Greek in the Philadelphia High School. He had by then published several books and after the trip to France, he published one in America, *Sketches in Paris* which was later republished in London as *The American in Paris.*

It was during this visit to Paris in 1835-6 that Dr James Stratton Carpenter, his son-in-law, travelled to Paris and London.

Following the trip to London, Dr James Stratton Carpenter returned to Pottsville to resume his practice, which he continued with success until his death in 1872. His reputation for great skill extended far beyond the limits of his practice.   He helped organise the Schuylkill Medical Society in 1845, three years before the Pennsylvania Medical Society was formed. He served as president of the state society in 1855.

The Carpenters had nine children.   The first son, of whom he speaks in his diary was John Thomas.   John Thomas was born June 17th 1833, in Pottsville, Pennsylvania and attended the Pottsville Academy. He graduated from the University of Pennsylvania in 1852 and the medical college of the same institution in 1855. He started practice in Pottsville, but soon joined the Pennsylvania reserves. He served in various capacities during the Civil War: as Medical Director in hospitals in Cumberland, Maryland; Cincinnati, Ohio; as Medical Director of the Department of Ohio; as Medical Director and Superintendent of Hospitals in the District of Ohio, and as President of the Army Medical Board. Later he was President of the Medical Society of Pennsylvania in 1880.

He married Elizabeth Adelaide Hill in 1855, and after her death, the widow of General Henry Pleasants.   There were ten children by the first marriage, including James Stratton Carpenter II who was born in 1859.

James Stratton Carpenter II was also born in Pottsville.   He graduated from Trinity College in 1879 and received his MD from the University of Pennsylvania in 1882.   Following this he served as Resident Physician in the Episcopal Hospital of Philadelphia, from 1882-83. James Stratton II also practised in Pottsville, Pennsylvania, until his death in 1920. He married Lillian Louise Chapin in 1886 and they had four children. Dr Carpenter was the author of numerous papers, and served as an officer in the Pennsylvania National Guard for a number of years. In 1916 he was joined in medical practice by his first son, Dr James Carpenter III.

The last of the four Carpenter doctors to practice medicine in Pottsville was born in 1887 and attended Trinity College like his father in 1908, and the University of Pennsylvania Medical College in 1913. Following an internship at the University of Pennsylvania Hospital, he started his medical career in Pottsville, which was interrupted for a short time by service in the Army during the Mexican Border dispute, but on returning to his native city, he practised medicine there until 1969. During his long life, he served as President of the Schuylkill County Medical Society, was Chief of Medical Services at the Pottsville Hospital for twenty-nine years and a member of the staff of both Pottsville hospitals. He was regional physician for the Pennsylvania Railroad for forty years and a lifetime member of Trinity Episcopal Church, Pottsville where he was vestryman and senior warden for some period of time.

Dr Carpenter married Clare Dechert, daughter of a Schuylkill Haven physician, in 1916. They had four children: James Stratton Carpenter IV, Daniel Dechert Carpenter, Peter Carpenter and the co-editor of this diary, Cornelia Carpenter Ferguson.

A Brief History Of London

'I fell in love with London at first sight when I arrived there... in the late spring of 1922, and have been in love with it ever since.'
John Gunther, at the age of twenty.

'When a man is tired of London, he is tired of life; for there is in London all that life can afford.'
Dr Samuel Johnson.

'Dear, damn'd, distracting town.'
Alexander Pope.

'The citizens of London are noted above all other citizens for the elegance of their manners, dress, table and discourse.'
Thomas Beckett, in the twelfth century.

Although Dr James Stratton Carpenter does not express his love for London in such brief eloquent words, the following diary shows that he enjoyed the city for the six months he was there in 1836. To many generations of Americans, London was the greatest city in the world, and for years it was listed as the largest city in the world.[1] Today, with a population of nearly seven million, it is smaller than New York City, Cairo, Calcutta, Canton, Jakarta, Mexico City, Peking, Sao Paulo, Shanghai, Tokyo and perhaps several other cities. Paris, where Dr James had spent six months prior to going to London, was only about one third the size of London by today's figures.

The Romans probably chose the site of London in about the year AD43, on the north bank of the river Thames, approximately sixty

---

[1] See page 94 of the diary for information on the size and geography of London.

miles from the sea. There is no documentation as to an earlier occupation and fortification, but after Caesar's invasion, markets and commerce quickly began to grow.

There was a native rebellion in 301 AD which the Romans quickly put down and they almost immediately began to fortify the city with a great wall, which stood until the fire of 1666. This wall was twenty feet high, eight feet thick, over two miles long and it enclosed an area of nearly four hundred acres for fourteen centuries, enclosing virtually the entire city. Some of the gates have a familiar ring today: Bishopsgate, Aldgate, and Newgate.

A number of builders, for example Emperor Theodosius or Constantine, were credited with the building of the wall which was completed several hundred years later.

There is little information and disagreement concerning the London of the Dark Ages (409-884 AD), but the Romans withdrew and there were invasions from the Anglo Saxons and the Vikings.

Between 889 and 1066, Alfred the Great restored London, rebuilt the wall, organised a government, restored the Navy, developed education with the founding of University College, Oxford, and developed trade and commerce. Christianity had come to London earlier, and although it was not become a strong influence, it was still alive.

The Norman Conquest and subsequent government, 1066-1154, brought new life to the city and also great change. More substantial buildings replaced the rather primitive structures of the earlier times. It was during this period that the first Tower of London was built. Areas familiar today began to develop, such as the market area at Cheapside, and a replacement for the early London Bridge. The building of churches started, including St Paul's which would take several hundred years to complete.

During the period from 1154 to 1485, London grew at a fast pace and became one of the great cities of mediaeval Europe with more than one hundred craft guilds. Its wharves were piled high with goods of trade and its waterways were crowded with vessels from throughout Europe.

The Magna Carta of 1215 paved the way for constitutional monarchy by recognising that a king could be bound by laws enforceable by his subjects. The Crusades of 1095-1254 broadened the horizons of the British by developing a more international attitude.

This was the age of Chaucer, the first great English poet: his *Troilus and Criseyde* and *Canterbury Tales*, established his reputation. Up until this time, French had been the official language of the Parliament and law courts.

Religious life was at full pace by this stage in England and saw the phenomena of preaching friars. There were the Black Friars, the Grey Friars, the Austin Friars, the White Friars and many others. Thomas Becket wrote in his eulogy of the City of London that in addition to St Paul's Cathedral, there were thirteen other large churches and over a hundred small parish churches.

It was during this period that Westminster Abbey was built, 1245-1260 and upon which Henry III lavished both money and gifts.

London was now a city of beautiful large churches, palaces and homes built of stone. It was a busy noisy city which conducted considerable commerce with Europe.

As London moved into the Tudor age, 1485-1603, it left the mediaeval age behind and moved into a more vigorous period. Three events were to influence the city: its people and the monarchs. The Reformation, the Renaissance, which started in Italy and moved up across Europe, and the discovery of America.

The Tudors were of Welsh descent. Henry Tudor, Earl of Richmond, ended the War of Roses in 1485 and became Henry VII. He was succeeded by the well known Henry VIII (1509-47), Edward VI, Mary I and Elizabeth I. England became a major world power.

The numerous monasteries and convents were to a great extent destroyed, and many of the children, the sick and the aged were put into the streets. This resulted in the first of the royal hospitals. This dismal condition in London was overshadowed by the discovery of America and a new route to India. This was the age of Shakespeare (1564-1616). London became a world capital and the chief commercial city of Europe. Others who aided in the growing reputation of London were Sir Francis Drake (1543-1596), the first Englishman to sail around the world, who later destroyed or dispersed the Spanish Armada; Sir Walter Raleigh (1554-1618) poet adventurer; Francis Bacon (1561-1626) a philosopher who became Lord Chancellor to James I, but is remembered for his stimulus to scientific research in England; and Christopher Marlowe (1564-1593) the poet dramatists, a major influence on Shakespeare and many other writers of the period.

London of the seventeenth century was a time of political difficulty and also the era of Samuel Pepys. The bubonic plague killed over 75,000 people. The fire of 1666 destroyed nearly all of the city: over four hundred acres were in ruins and more than thirteen thousand homes had burned, leaving more than two hundred thousand people homeless. This necessitated a complete rebuilding of the city. Fortunately, Sir Christopher Wren (1632-1723), the greatest of English architects, was coming into his prime, He turned to architecture in 1663, having taught himself as he had been trained as a mathematician and astronomer. After the fire he was appointed the principal architect to rebuild London – an awesome responsibility since this included fifty-two churches, government buildings and a new master plan for the city. His greatest building was undoubtedly St Paul's Cathedral, but other buildings such as the Greenwich buildings and the hospital in Chelsea were very handsome. Although Wren's plan for the city was not carried out to any great extent, he can be credited with changing the appearance of London. The individual citizens started rebuilding their homes immediately on the ruins of their former dwellings, thus preserving the old plan of curving streets with the same names.

The city also grew, spreading westward. Commercially, the incorporation of the Bank of England during this period was most significant.

Eighteenth century London, changed the geography of the city by further westward movement with the development of such well known squares as Grosvenor, Cavendish and Hanover. Samuel Johnson, writer, poet, essayist and newspaperman, gives us a view of the vice and corruption of the day which was painted by Hogarth in *The Rake's Progress*. Johnson also described the many changes in the city, such as the demolishing of some of the gates of the old wall, the tearing down of houses which lined London Bridge, the increase in commerce and trade and the sociability of the city.

The defeat of Napoleon at the battle of Waterloo in 1815 by the Anglo-Dutch army under the English General, Wellington, and the sinking or capture of the French-Spanish fleet by Admiral Nelson, ushered in the nineteenth century. Great Britain had a fast increasing total population of thirteen million[2] which would double before the end of the century.

The period 1830-1850 was the era of railways steamships and gas lights in Britain. During the time Dr James Carpenter was in London, more than thirty-nine bills were passed, adding new lines to British railways, (fifty-four had been passed in 1835), and adding more than one thousand miles of railroads. These lines provided a need as well as a means of transportation for the tremendous increase in coal and iron output in the 1830s. Another important act which was passed at this time was the law which prohibited child labour; no child under eleven, (1833), twelve the next year and thirteen the following year could be employed more than forty-eight hours a week, or more than nine in one day.

Although the London of 1836 was spreading rapidly in all directions, the heart of the city remained as it is today: no larger than that of Roman times. This was the London of Charles Dickens (1812-1870) who was a young writer in 1836 and was probably writing *The Pickwick Papers* (1837). in his spare time

William IV (1830-1837) was the king during Carpenter's visit to London. He is known as the 'Sailor King' as he had served at sea from the age of fifteen, starting as an 'able seaman', and although unassuming and not over-intelligent, he was capable and possessed of some statesmanlike qualities, which he exhibited as king from 1830-1837. King William was noted for his informal ways and for his embarrassing candour. He had no surviving issue by his queen, Adelaide, daughter of the Duke of Saxe-Coburn and Meiningen, with whom he lived happily for many years. He was succeeded by his late brother's daughter, Princess Victoria of Kent.

---

[2] See page 94 of the diary for the population of London in 1836

In the course of the editing of this diary, no alteration was made to the spelling, punctuation or grammar of the original text. Information concerning medical practice, however, was eliminated.

Diary Of Dr James Stratton Carpenter

7 Sacksville Street[3]
Piccadilly, London   July 18, 1836

July 17, Sunday – Put on a case of scrotal hernia,[4] the first in London. German about twenty-eight years of age – pays ten pounds[5] in advance and ten more when cured.

Rode out on the top of a coach to Hounslow.[6] Hounslow heath so celebrated in story and in the annals of highway

---

[3] Located about three short blocks from Piccadilly Circus, as early as 1596 the area was named for a flower, Pickadilla. Today Sacksville Street is an attractive area just off of Regent Street, and the home of a number of speciality shops, including a shirtmaker at No.7 and a rare bookshop nearby. The Royal Academy of Arts (Burlington House), on Piccadilly Street is at the west end of the next block and an Underground Station is about the same distance to the east. St James Church (1684) designed by Sir Christopher Wren, is just around the corner on from Sacksville Street. Seriously damaged in World War II, it was restored in 1954.

A number of well known personalities resided on this street prior to JSC's visit: Charles Kemble the actor, at number 5 in 1819; Lord Bloomfield at number 6 in 1829; Lt. Colonel Robert Torrens, a political economist, at number 7 in 1813 and Sir Gilbert Blane, a celebrated Naval Physician, at number 8 in 1831.

[4] A hernia is a swelling or bulge of tissue which protrudes through the abdominal muscles or area of the reproductive organs. Today hernias are usually repaired by surgery.

[5] Approximately forty-five dollars in 1836.

robbery, has been enclosed and put under cultivation. Excepting six hundred acres, which has been reserved for a parade ground. This heath which formerly produced nothing but fern and Poverty grass, was a common, but by an act of Parliament was divided among the freeholders in that parish or neighbourhood who possessed the right of common. The village of Hounslow which contains... inhabitants is a neat place, possesses a very neat church. Passed through Kensington,[7] Brentford and some other small places. In returning passed through Wickham. Richmond[8] commands a most beautiful prospect of the Thames as it winds through the rich meadows and among the old oaks, the pride of England – and numerous county seats.

Distance from London to Hounslow ten miles fare 2 S.[9] The seat of Lord Holland[10] on the road to Richmond is a fine old building, with a noble park attached to it. Turnham Green 5 miles from London, near which are the horticultural gardens, is

---

[6] Hounslow, see the next page of the diary. The 'Coach', or omnibus, had been introduced in 1829, but was horse drawn. To a great extent railroads replaced stagecoaches during the 1840's.

[7] Kensington in the early nineteenth century was transformed from a rural parish of less than ten thousand inhabitants, to over two hundred thousand by the end of the century. Originally, Kensington Gardens were attached to Nottingham House which was bought by William III and converted into Kensington Palace by Sir Christopher Wren. It has been the home of a number of English monarchs. Four members of the Royal family who died in this palace were Mary II, William III, Anne, and George III. Queen Victoria was born at Kensington in 1819 and lived there until she ascended to the throne in 1837.

[8] Originally, Richmond on the Thames was a village of fishermen's cottages.

[9] At this time, a shilling (twenty per pound) was probably worth about forty-six cents.

[10] His lordship's house at Kensington was, for a very long period, a hospitable resort for those distinguished in literature and politics. He died at Holland House in 1840.

a little village with nothing important and I only mention it in connection with the gardens. There are three exhibitions held here annually, to which all the world of fashion flock, because it is fashionable, there being nothing very remarkable to see in itself.

Monday, July 18 – Wrote to Camilla[11] and a letter of seven pages and half to Thomas, and put them in the bag at the coffee house.

Paid *The Standard* (London Newspaper) 1 pound 10 ($6.80) for five insertions of my advertisement to be put in every other day and 6S ($1.20) to insert a notice of my 'Remarks' – visited *The Times*,[12] *Morning Herald* and *John Bull*.[13]

Read Mrs Trollope's, *Jonathan Jefferson Whitlow*.[14] It is a description of a certain portion of our south. Slave holding

---

[11] Camilla was JSC's wife, living in Pottsville, Pennsylvania. She was the daughter of John and Sophie Sanderson and the mother of two children, John Thomas (June 1833) and Sarah Stratton (June 1835). The 'half page' letter was undoubtedly addressed to his three year old son Thomas.

[12] An 'Insertion' from *The Times* (September 15, 1836), *The Standard* (July 21, 1836), and *John Bull* (August 7, 1836):
'RADICAL CURE of HERNIA or RUPTURE, by the new American method, in from 20 to 40 days without operation, and unattended by pain or interruption of business. The approbation of the faculty of Philadelphia, and more than 200 cases cured, attest the efficacy of this plan. It is applicable to every variety of Rupture, to both sexes and all ages. Just published (a pamphlet), price 1S. Remarks on the Radical Cure of Rupture, with testimonials of Faculty, etc. By JS Carpenter, M.D. Effingham Wilson, 88 Royal Exchange; and H. Bickers, 1, Leicester Square. Dr. Carpenter may be consulted every day from 10 till 3 at 7, Sacksville Street, Piccadilly.'

[13] See pages 98-100 for JSC's evaluation of London Newspapers.

[14] Mrs Trollope (Frances) 1780-1863, was married to the author Thomas Anthony Trollope. They were in America during the late 1820s. Her husband (with the family of five children) tried to farm

population, caricatures – with a good many misrepresentations and many slanders. She had a goodly stock of venom, all of which she seems desirous of pouring upon the heads of the Americans.

Thursday, July 21 – I have made a rule of writing and reading French every day for a couple of hours, that I may not loose, what I have already gained & that I may improve my self in the grammatical construction of the language.[15] Read N.P. Willis' *Inklings of Adventure*.[16] Many of the descriptions awful, and some of the incidents highly interesting and

---

near Cincinnati, Ohio. Unhappily this plan did not succeed, and the family returned to England in 1830. With a need to support her family Mrs Trollope wrote and published in 1832, *Domestic Manners of the Americans*. The book was not popular in America, because of her very critical remarks, especially about slavery. Mrs Trollope was a prolific writer and traveller.

[15] John Sanderson, the father-in-law, was in Paris from June 1835 until early fall of 1836, and although he published two books, there is no reference to his son-in-law; however, he used the pronoun 'we' frequently. *Familiar Letters to Friends* (1838) and a two volume work, *The American in Paris* were the two books. The father-in-law was a teacher as well as writer so it is easy to assume both men learned to read and write French.

[16] NP Willis 1806-1867 was a journalist, poet, editor and dramatist born in Maine of a family of journalists. He graduated from Yale in 1827 and at twenty-three established *American Monthly Magazine* in Boston which was successful for several years. He then went to New York where he was associated with *The Mirror* which sent him abroad for five years as a foreign correspondent. Willis was adored by English society. One lady described him as 'More like one of the best of our peer's sons than a rough republican'. He returned to America with an English bride in 1836, but returned to England several times later. He was always a pet of society and a popular magazine writer. His book, *Inklings of Adventure* which JSC read, was first published in 1836.

sometimes amusing – but they are generally frothy, light as a syllabi and like it – agreeable without much substance.

Friday, July 22 – Recd. a letter from Dr Tucker[17] in which he says that Dr Baigly has written an article for them of considerable length and will send it to me. Mr Ewing has also written a letter in attestation of his cure. Recd. a letter from my dear Camilla (via Paris) dated June 11 P.V. – wants me to send her some French worked capes and collars – chintzy & drapes – etc – Oh! how I long to see my beloved family – surely if there not be happiness in the society of a wife who loves me and of children lovely as the angels of light who look up to me as their father and protector, it is not to be found elsewhere.

Mr Smith, 44 Paradise Row, Chelsea,[18] has sent for me, for the purpose of consulting me on a type of hernia that he has.

Paid *Times* three pounds to insert my announce ten times. *Monsieur mon malade* called – *il va bien pour le temps.*

---

[17] A letter from the French Patent Office (Institut National De La Propriete Industrielle) dated '19 Avr. 91' contains the following:

'James Stratton Carpenter.

Patent Certificate of introduction and of perfection of ten years taken October 31, 1835. 'System of hernia bandages to the aid of which one wants, when the reduction is possible, to operate the radical cure of all hernias.'

'I signal you that Mr Carpenter, owner of this diploma, gave up May 23, 1836 all his rights to (Dr) Herisson and (Dr) Tucker who were at the time doctors in Paris.'

There are several mentions in the diary concerning these two French doctors.

[18] There is a Paradise Walk in Chelsea one block from the Royal Hospital. Number 44 is a modern building occupied by an architectural firm, but the remainder of the area is a row of small homes.

20

Saturday, July 23 – Received a certificate from Dr A.B. Tucker & one from M. Le Docteur Herisson, the latter highly complimentary of my personal ability.

Rode up to Chelsea and visited Mr Smith, at 87. Advised him not to attempt a cure, for which he paid me a guinea. One that he had hoarded up in his youth. There are but very few of that coin in circulation – only to be found in the possession of sexagenarians and antiquarians.

Chelsea, situated on the Thames, about three miles above London, is now almost joined and incorporated in the all absorbing gulf of this vast metropolis. It is principally noted for an extensive hospital for old and disabled soldiers, and the beautiful gardens & grounds attached It was founded by Charles 2nd, but great improvements & additions have since been made – the chapel is a fine long & lofty room hung with the flags of different nations, taken in battle, among which was several bearing the imperial eagle and the name of Napoleon. The Stars and Stripes of my own country were not absent – but I think the English have no cause of boasting on that subject. If our eagle has sometimes been put to flight, the British Lion has been sent growling and discomforted back to his island den, more than once. The dining-room corresponds in size & decorations with the chapel, and occupies the half of the same building. I passed through the wards and was gratified with the cleanliness, neatness and comfort which appears to reign there – each man has his bed & his birth opening into the long, common hall or passage.[19]

---

[19] A plaque on the main building at the Royal Hospital reads as follows:

'For the succour and relief of aged veterans and men broken by war, founded by Charles II, enlarged by James II, completed by William and Mary, King and Queen in the year of our Lord 1692.'

The building was designed by Sir Christopher Wren. The cost was approximately one hundred fifty thousand pounds ($675,000). At the time JSC visited Chelsea, it was being enlarged by Sir John Sloane

Sunday, July 24th – I dined yesterday at Chelsea and had simply a mutton chop, bread & a pint of ale. The ale was apparently very fine 'clear as crystal, pure as amber & strong and brandy' but it produced first a dryness, then a drowsiness, a parched throat & headache, sleeplessness, great thirst, loss of appetite, a burning in the throat, bad taste in the mouth, thick, high colored urine, etc. In fact a gastritis which did not go off for two days. I believe the ale had in it an unusual quantity of coculus indicus – a poisonous 'berry' added to the ale to make it heady.

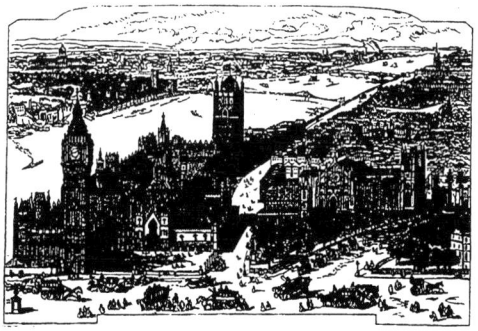

Houses of Parliament, Westminster Abbey, Westminster Hall, Crimean and Canning Monuments

Westminster Abbey[20] – Attended church this afternoon in this time honoured building. What an admirable structure such

---

who was responsible for the design of some of the small buildings on the either sides of the main building. There was considerable damage by bombs in 1941 but restoration was completed by 1961.

Today, Chelsea is noted, in addition to the hospital, for the beautiful annual spring flower show held on the extensive lawn in front of the main buildings. There are also permanent gardens on site.

[20] The foundation for Westminster Abbey was laid by St Sebert, the Confessor. The original buildings were a monastery and for over 700 years, there were monks at Westminster. The great eleventh century

lightness, & elegance, combined with strength and durability. How much time, & labour and money must have been lavished upon it. It is remarkable not only for the vastness of size & beauty of architecture, but still more from the great events connected with its history and the great names who lie entombed within its walls. As I stood under that high roof & listened to the pealing organ as it rolled down the long aisle and

---

church, which replaced an earlier and more primitive edifice, was built under the personal direction of Edward the Confessor. This early church in turn was replaced by the present Abbey Church which was built between 1245 and 1269. Henry III lavished both money and gifts. Building the Norman nave received financial help from both Richard II and Henry V. Henry VII raised funds to add a chapel which was built in a perpendicular style by skilled architects and sculptors. This splendid chapel bears his name. After the final dissolution of the monastery, Queen Elizabeth I established the present Collegiate Church. No further additions were made until the two western towers were completed in 1745, during the reign of William and Mary, who had the entire abbey repaired and the towers, designed by Sir Christopher Wren, were added (Nicholas Hawksmoor and John James were the actual architects of the two towers).

The length of the abbey is 416 feet; width at the transept, 203 feet; at the nave, 102 feet; and the height of the west towers is 225 feet.

The Chapter House, started by Henry II, became the meeting place for the House of Commons in the mid 13th Century and continued until the time of Henry VIII. The first burials within the Abbey were confined to sovereigns, members of the Royal Family, abbots of the monastery, and a few royal favourites. However, by the 16th century burials became more common, and towering monuments were erected to some of the great Elizabethans, including poets and writers, musicians, etc. The names of persons buried in the Abbey reads like the Who's Who of England including many kings and queens, great poets, painters and others.

Washington Irving wrote, "Suddenly the notes of the deep-labouring organ burst upon the ear, falling with doubled and redoubled intensity, and rolling, as it were in huge billows of sound. How well do their volume and grandeur accord with this mighty building!"

among the arches & pillars – or the wild and unearthly sound of the chanters – I felt carried back to other days and as the sunbeams & shadows chased each other in rapid succession – from pillar to pillar – they seemed to me like the spirit of the place, the ghosts of departed days, wandering in their wonted familiar places. There is so much of romance as well of historical reminiscence in this place that my imagination wandered immediately that enter it, back among the dim records of ancient times. I seemed to converse with the mighty dead whose ashes and monuments are around & below me.

Monday, July 25 – read James's new novel, 3 Vols *One and a Thousand, or Days of Henri Quatre.*[21] I think it is decidedly inferior to most if not all of his previous productions, not only in interest of plot, but description of scenery & characters. Still, I believe it a correct idea of the manners of the times and throws some light on the characters of some of the principle actors of the days of Henry the fourth.

Looked over Tait's *Edinburgh Magazine* July 1836[22]. A rich man, or he has great merit being the autobiography of

---

[21] George Payne Rainsford James (1801-1860) wrote *One and a Thousand, or the Days of Henri Vingt-Quatre*, a novel of the League (1589-90) taking up the story of the religious wars just before the murder of Henry III and a careful study of the history and portrait of Henry IV. Sir Walter Raleigh and Washington Irving were his mentors. Because of his success as a writer, particularly historical, he was appointed historiographer of England by William IV, but soon resigned to become British Consul to Virginia in 1852. He continued writing and publishing while in America. James was sent to Venice afterwards as Consul-General where he died in 1860. His biographer does not mention the book read by JSC.

[22] *Tait's Magazine* for July 1836 contained a number of interesting articles including, 'Tours 7 Detours in Scotland' written by a family; 'Principles of Morality of the People called Quakers' by Wm Howitt, (JSC's great, great, great, grandfather, a Quaker, came to America and settled in the Philadelphia colony with William Penn; 'A Rich

Archibald Plack, late Lord Mayor of London, is excellent – written in Galt's[23] best style – full of humour and satire – Basil Hall[24] *Schoss Wainfield or a Winter in Lower Syria* contains some interesting circumstances connected with the early career of Sir Walter Scott. Miss Jane Ann Cranstoun married Count Purystall, original of Die Vernon.

Tuesday, July 26th – Mr Eccles[25] called.

Went with Messrs Sybert and Sanderson and Dr(no name) of the Navy of the US, to Greenwich – starting from London Bridge,[26] we walked about a mile along the line of arches which

---

Man' – the autobiography of the late Lord Mayor of London by John Galt (continued from the June issue); Captain Basil Hall's 'Schloss Hainfield or a Winter in Lower Syria' and a Literary Bulletin for July, a political Register, and 'Postscripts'.

[23] Galt, a Scotsman who started as a businessman, the study of law, and for a time an emigration agent in Canada, became a prolific writer.

[24] Captain and Mrs Basil Hall had visited America in 1828 and both published their writings. Basil was quite complimentary in most cases, especially concerning the plantations he visited on Coastal Georgia. Mrs Hall was not always so kind.

[25] Two Eccles are mentioned frequently, Mr George a printer-engraver and his brother Walter Eccles, a surgeon, listed as a member of the Royal College of Surgeons, 1824-1838. Mr George Eccles may have produced the brochure which Dr C distributed.

[26] The first London bridge was probably built by the Romans in the early tenth century. Many Roman coins were discovered in the ruins of this early bridge when a medieval bridge (1176) was demolished and replaced by a stone structure of twenty arches, which had a row of houses on each side. Many of these houses were burned in 1213. The bridge was over nine hundred feet long. However, the number of piers were a serious handicap to navigation. An old proverb says that the bridge was made "for wise men to go over, and fools to go under."

A new bridge was built and opened with great ceremony by the King and Queen in 1831. It was 928 feet long, 54 feet wide, and had 5

support this road to where it is finished and got into the carriage drawn by a locomotive, we rode by two miles, and walked the rest of the way – about a mile – Greenwich[27] is celebrated on account of its Hospital for infirm and disabled seaman. It is a

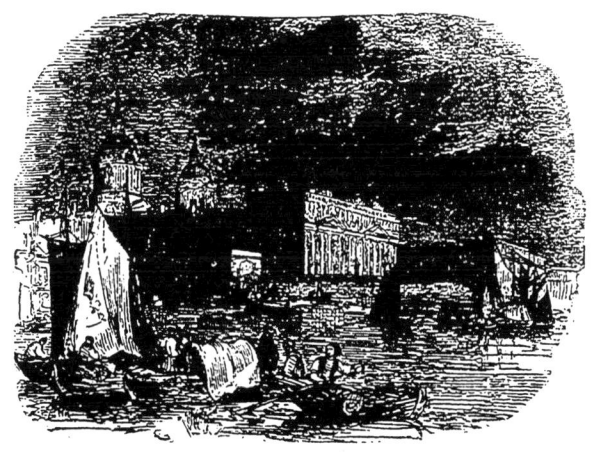

Greenwich

noble building and with its beautiful Italian portico, and double domes, has a fine effect particularly from the river on the bank

---

arches of which the centre arches were 152 feet. This bridge was regarded as one of the finest granite bridges in the world, and was the bridge which JSC crossed. When the present bridge was built in 1968 the earlier bridge was moved piece by piece to the desert of Arizona in America over Lake Havasu.

[27] Greenwich is six miles from London – four miles from the London Bridge, a few minutes by train today or a pleasant ride by boat. Greenwich has handsome buildings designed by Sir Christopher Wren and Indigo Jones. William and Mary established the hospital in 1694 for old and disabled seaman. Today the buildings have different uses than described by JSC. One of the large rooms is now a beautiful dining-hall; the paintings he mentions are still on view, but at different locations.

of which it is built – the western dome is occupied as a naval gallery of paintings and statues and models of ships etc. A great number of portraits of naval heroes adorn the walls some of them sufficiently bad paintings – the ceilings are covered with allegorical figures, etc. An astrolabe,[28] formerly belonging to Sir Francis Drake, and the coat which Nelson wore at the Battle of Trafalgar, enclosed in a box with a glass cover, & much moth eaten were the principal objects of curiosity. In the opposite dome, occupied as a chapel there is nothing remarkable – it is neat commodious room, with a painting of the shipwreck of Paul on the island of Milletus – the serpent which bit St Paul is hanging on his hand and the cane is illuminated by the fire which had been built. A neat monument near the door erected by William IV to the memory of his watchmate and messmate, Admiral Keats (I think) shows that the sailor king is not ashamed of his having been a midshipman.

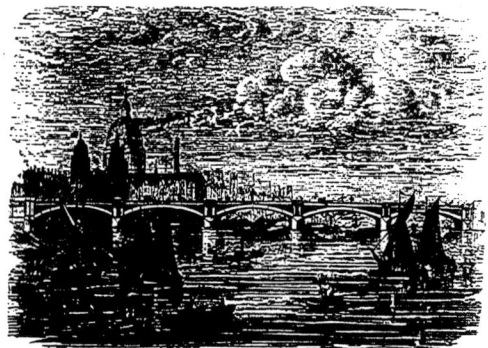

Blackfriars Bridge

---

[28] An Astrolabe was a compact instrument used to observe and calculate the position of celestial bodies before the invention of the sextant and is on view in the observatory up the hill where it is possible to place one foot in one time zone and the other foot in another time zone. The Nelson coat is still on display, although there is some doubt about its authenticity.

We dined at the Royal George Tavern, on the edge of the river, and were surprised with a good dinner – for from the external appearance of the house we did not expect much. Returning we took the steam boat[29] to Hungerford market, and passed under the noble bridges which span old father Thames – New London Bridge, southward Blackfriars[30] and Waterloo bridges[31] – Westminster Bridge[32] comes next and lastly Vauxhall.[33] Hungerford market[34] where we landed is a Pretty building lately erected. The manner in which they continue to expose the fish to the open air, and yet keep them fresh is

---

[29] 1830-1850 was the era of steam boats and steam railroads, James Watts had developed the steam engine in the late 18th century and Robert Fulton applied steam to boats early in the 19th century.

[30] Blackfriars Bridge, which JSC saw, was built in 1769 as designed by Robert Mylne at a cost of 152,840 pounds. It had nineteen arches and was 995 long. The replacement bridge was opened by Queen Victoria in 1860, and was much wider and over twelve hundred feet long with a span of 185 feet at the centre to permit river traffic

[31] Waterloo Bridge, made of Scottish granite, was opened for the 2nd anniversary of the Battle of Waterloo in 1817, after six years of construction. John Rennie was the designer and the cost was one million pounds. The bridge rested on three hundred and twenty piers driven into the river. During World War II, the bridge was damaged and in addition to deterioration, one of the finest bridges was extensively repaired

[32] Westminster Bridge was built 1739-1750 by a Swiss named Labelyeat at a cost of four hundred thousand pounds (over one and three quarters million dollars). This bridge started a trend in bridge building (completely level) and remained one of the handsomest until 1881, when the present bridge near the Parliament was built.

[33] Vauxhall Bridge was an iron bridge which had opened in 1816 at a cost of only a hundred and fifty thousand pounds. The designer was James Walker. Today's bridge was built in 1890.

[34] The Hungerford Market was built in 1682 and rebuilt in 1833 just before JSC arrived in London. The market had two floors of stalls for selling meat, fish, fruit and vegetables. In 1860 it was demolished to make way for Charing Cross Railroad Station.

worthy of notice. They are laid on white slabs of marble, raised one above another like a steps of a porch, and a constant stream of clean fresh water kept running over them. Wednesday, July 27 Mr H. Bickers sent for some more of my pamphlets having sold the first dozen – I sent him thirteen more.

Called at the office of *The Sunday Times* to inquire after my advertisement, I was told that the man who called here to solicit the insertion of my announce was a cheat, that they had no person so employed, that it was a 'do' – 5 shillings ($1.15) is not very high to pay for a little experience.

Went to a Grand Gala at the Vauxhall Gardens[35] with Mr Sybert and Dr H – met Professor Hare of Philadelphia. The gardens were lit up with tens of thousands of variegated lamps – interspersed amongst grass hung in festoons around the trees. Rotunda covered with them, in which were placed the musicians. Italian walk adorned with statues – at the upper end of which was a fine view of the city and bay of Naples. Ballet - rope dancing – fireworks & music constituted the amusements of the evening.

Thursday, July 28th – Read the first volume of the *Diary of a Desennuyee*[36] – treats of the manners of high life in London, and if the portrait drawn by the authoress is correct, which it is said to be the people of fashion and rank are not much to be envied even by the lowest class of people. From her it appears that they are frivolous, weak minded and contemptible to the

---

[35] The exceptionally beautiful Vauxhall Gardens, 1660 to 1859, were located across the Thames in the area of the present day Tate Gallery. In 1836 the gardens were frequently referred to by writers like Pepys, Fielding, and others. The name derives from Fox Hall by a variety of spellings. There were lighted walks, gardens, areas for dancing and for celebrating events such as the Battle of Waterloo.

[36] [Catherine Grace Frances (Moody) Gore], *The Diary of a Desennuyee* 2 Vols. (London: H. Colburn, 1836).

highest degree. The book is written with great deal of spirit, and the authoress must have moved in the scenes which she describes so graphically.

Read the new monthly magazine for July 1836 *The Sirens and Mermaids* – 'Delicate Attentions' 'Steeple Hunting' are the principle articles – Mr Sergeant Talfourd's[37] tragedy of ION highly commended. Mr Landon[38] also called *The Death of Clytemnestra* yet unpublished is puffed in advance – *Liberty and Slavery in America* (Misrepresented both).

Friday, July 29, 1836 – Wrote to Camilla – Read second volume of the *Desennuyee* which give us a peep at the Tuileries and French society, which I think is very correct, at least as far as my observation goes. She speaks of Trollope and her works on Frances the MD with a good deal of contempt – called her Goody Trollope.

Saturday, July 30th – A great special beauty of London is the numbering of squares[39] not like the places in Paris, paved

---

[37] Sir Thomas Talfourd was a member of Parliament when JSC was reading his play, ION, produced at Covent Garden, perhaps after JSC returned to America. Talfourd was a contributor to *New Monthly Magazine*, *Edinburgh* and the *Quarterly*. He was loved and respected both as a writer, a judge and as a member of Parliament.

[38] This may be a reference to Walter Savage Landon, a modern English poet, essayist and writer who contributed to magazines in the first half of the nineteenth century. His *Letters of an American* was published under a pseudonym, but not until long after JSC returned home.

[39] Back in JSC's day, the mass of streets west of the crossing of Oxford and Regent streets were mostly private residences, such as St James, Hanover, Berkeley, Grosvenor, Cavendish, Bryanstone, Manchester and Portman Squares.

The residences of Berkeley Square, one of the most aristocratic, included Horace Walpole, William Pitt and Beau Brummell.

Gough Square (Fleet Street), No. 17 was the home of Dr Johnson.

with stones, but enclosed with elegant Iron railings, planted with trees, flowers and shrubs and the fine green turf intersected with gravel walks. They are however, only open to the families who live around them.

The view down the Thames from London Bridge is peculiarly striking. What a forest of masts, and what ceaseless activity! Compared with this, Paris is nothing, with its half dozen Seine boats and one bit of a steamboat – on the other hand, here is a total want of the magnificent quays which border the Seine from one end of Paris to the other and are its chief ornament.[40]

Sunday, July 31st – Accompanied by Mr Sanderson, Dr H and Mr Sybert, started this morning from the White Horse,

---

Grosvenor Square was originally laid out in 1695: some of the original ironwork is still visible on some of the houses. In 1895 the home of Lord Randolph Churchill was No. 50.

Hyde Park was originally the home of Westminster monks from the Norman Conquest until the time of Henry VIII. Today it is a busy area of London with a triple gate, the entrance to Hyde Park.

Leicester Square was home to four famous people, commemorated by statues in the gardens: Hogarth, Reynolds, Newton and John Hunter. The gardens in this very busy area were once a location for duels. It is still a busy area of theatres, restaurants, shops and a small booth with theatre tickets available at discount prices.

Trafalgar Square, named for Nelson's last victory, might have been under construction when JSC was in London.

[40] The Thames was filled with steamboats to take passengers between the many bridges, and presumably in JSC's day there were many ships delivering fish, vegetables and goods from abroad. The Thames Embankment as it is seen today was a vision of Sir Christopher Wren back in 1666, but it was not built until 1862. Embankment walks extended from the Westminster Bridge to Vauxhall and from Westminster Bridge to Blackfriars Bridge. Today they extend an even greater distance along the Thames.

Piccadilly, to visit Hampton Court,[41] the celebrated palace built by Cardinal Woolsey – it stands on the northern banks of the Thames about twelve miles due west from Hyde Park Corner. It was commenced about 1515, when finished, the building was

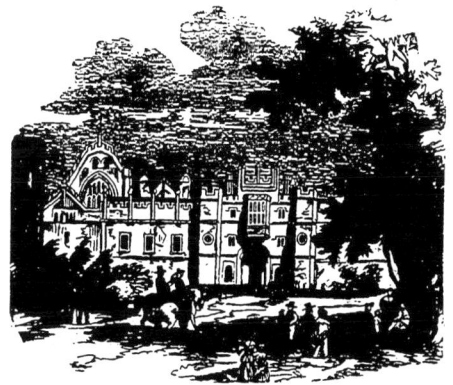

Hampton Court

in so magnificent a style that it began to excite great envy at Court. The King asked the Cardinal what were his intentions in building a palace that far surpassed any of the royal palaces of England – Woolsey, very politic replied, 'that he was only trying to form a residence worthy of so great a monarch' and that Hampton Court palace was the Property of the King Henry VIII which 'gained him much favour', Woolsey lived here in

---

[41] Cardinal Wolsey started Hampton Court Palace in 1514, but from 1525-1760 it was a Royal residence. In the late seventeenth century, Sir Christopher Wren was commissioned to enlarge the house; the principal facade seen today dates from that time. The palace was a favourite country residence of Henry VIII, who played tennis and jousted in its gardens. Five of his wives, including Seymour and Catherine Howard, are said to inhabit (as ghosts) the house. A fire in 1986 severely damaged some of the rooms of the state apartment created for William III and Queen Mary but these rooms have been carefully restored and reopened by the present Queen in July, 1992, however, this restoration does not always agree with the description of the apartments given by JSC in his diary of 1836.

more than regal state – this was his principal country residence, being Archbishop of York, Cardinal of... and Lord High Chancellor of England, he retained more than eight hundred persons in his suite. Edward VI was born in this palace his mother, Queen Jane Seymour, only survived his birth a few days. She was married to Henry VIII the day after the decapitation of the unfortunate Ann Boleyn, the 20th May 1536 and Edward VI was born 12th October 1537. Henry appears to have regarded this lady with more constancy and affection than any of his numerous wives, and seemed deeply affected at her death. Catherine Howard was the next Queen who figured here – after her the sixth wife was Lady Catherine Parr, sister of the Marquis Northampton and widow of Lord Latiner.

Queen Mary and Phillip[42] of Spain, her husband, passed their honeymoon in gloomy retirement at Hampton Court in 1558. Kept their Christmas here with great splendour. Elizabeth[43] becoming Queen, this Palace occasionally exhibited the same scenes of festivity, as in the days of Henry VIII. James I[44] took up his residence here soon after his arrival in England and on the 14th January 1603-4 began the celebrated conference between the Presbyterian and members of the established Church, held before King James as moderator and

---

[42] Queen Mary married Phillip, the son of Charles V of Spain. Queen Mary lived only a short time after the marriage.

[43] Elizabeth (daughter of Henry VIII) became Queen after the death of her sister Mary. Phillip of Spain offered to marry her and after considerable amount of coquetting, she declined. She reigned from 1558 until her death in 1603.

[44] James I, son of Henry Stuart (Lord Darnley) and Mary Queen of Scots, succeeded to the throne of Scotland when he was one year old (1567) and in 1603 to the throne of England following Queen Elizabeth. There were a number of plots to kill the king. He was a man of learning, especially in theology, writing a number of books on religious subjects. His adherence to the "divine right of kings" brought his son (Charles I) to the scaffold and led to the expulsion of the Stuarts from the English throne.

to it our omnipresent translation of the Bible. Queen Ann, the wife of James I died here 2 March 1618 and was interred in Westminster Abbey. In 1625 Charles I[45] and Queen Henrietta retired here to avoid the plagues of London. He was brought here by the Army in 1647 and kept in a state of imprisonment – until 11th November when he made his escape to the Isle of Wight – this was his favourite residence and he adorned its walls with many fine specimens of art, but they were scattered abroad by the round heads and they now form the choicest collections of foreign and private collections. Oliver Cromwell's daughter, Elizabeth[46] was married here to Lord Falconberg November 18, 1657 and the next year the Protectors witnessed there the death of his favourite daughter Mrs Claypole. Charles 2nd and James 2nd – resided there occasionally. On the abdication of the latter it became one of the favourite residences of William 3rd[47] – who made the palace what it now is, and laid out the gardens and park in their present form. Queen Mary his consort, was equally partial to this palace, and there is a bower of lime trees in the garden which still bears her name. George I[48] also sometimes held his

---

[45] Charles I, was the third son of James I and Anne. He was created Prince of Wales in 1616 and succeeded to the throne in 1625 and shortly married Henrietta Maria, daughter of Henry IV of France. He was executed on January 30, 1649. He had been a powerful and elegant writer, and was the father of Charles II and James II.

[46] Elizabeth, the third daughter of Oliver Cromwell, was a great talent and a great beauty.

[47] William III, son of William (Prince of Orange) and his wife Henrietta Marie, daughter of Charles I, married Princess Mary, daughter of James II. He took possession of the throne from Mary's father when he fled to France in 1689. William fell from his horse and was killed in 1702. His great aim was to curb the power of Louis XIV of France. It was the official apartment of William and Mary which was badly damaged in the fire of 1986.

[48] George I was created Duke of Cumberland in 1706 and succeeded Queen Anne to the throne in 1714. He died in 1727. He was said to

court here – the Great Hall was fitted up as a theatre and on the first October 1718. Henry VIII or the fall of Woolsey was represented on the very spot which had been the scene of his greatest splendour. Geo. 2nd[49] and his Queen Caroline were the last Sovereigns that resided at Hampton Court.

In its present state the Palace consists of three principal quadrangles – the western court is divided into several suites of apartments, occupied by private families. The middle quadrangle is called the Clock Court from a curious astronomical clock being placed over the gateway. Hampton Court was the first place where a public clock was put up in England.

The third quadrangle or Fountain Court was erected for King Wm 3rd by Sir C. Wren on the south side over the windows of the 12 labours of Hercules, in fresco, by Laquerne[50] and in the area is a *jet d'eau*. The western court is the only one which retains the original appearance. It is built of brick – the palace occupies eight acres of ground. In the fountain court on the north side is the Queen's staircase and southwest is a passage leading to the King's Grand Staircase, the ceilings and walls of which were painted by Verrio[51] a

---

have very simple tastes, and an unhappy marriage. His son George II succeeded him.

[49] George II succeeded his father in a period of great prosperity, with peace restored in 1729. However, there was a period of war again (1739-1748) against the Spanish and later in America (Canada was conquered). He died in the midst of glory in 1760.

[50] Louis Laquerne, a French painter, was the godson of Louis IV. He was taught by Le Brun and also at the Royal Academy in Paris. He came to England later and frequently painted ceilings, such as some in St Bartholomew's Hospital and later, at Hampton Court, the *Labours of Hercules*.

[51] Antonio Verrio was an Italian painter invited to England by Charles II to help decorate Windsor Castle. He also painted for James II and William III. He was associated with Laquerne at Hampton Court where he died in 1707.

Neapolitan painter brought to England by Chas. 2nd. It is crowded with allegories, richly ornamented with numerous devices in a most florid style. From the King's staircase, we entered the Guard Chamber, a magnificent room 60 x 37 and 30 feet high. The walls are covered with muskets, halberts, pistols, swords, drums and bandoliers, frontlets and daggers etc. arranged in various figures – there are sufficient equipment for a 1000 men. On the lower panels are some battle pieces. From the Guard's hall we entered the King's first presence Chamber. The walls are covered with Paintings Principally by Kneller,[52] among which are full length portraits of the beauties of William & Mary's Court & a picture of his landing at Torbay. These are all by that painter. The canopy of King Wm's throne still remains with the King's Arms and a Dutch Motto. The Third apartment is called the second presence chamber and is also adorned with numerous paintings by Van Dyke,[53] Veronese,[54] Sir J. Reynolds,[55] Titian,[56] and others The

---

[52] Kneller, Sir Godfrey was educated at Leyden for military service, but preferred to draw and paint. He studied under Rembrandt and later in Rome. When he visited in England, he quickly became well known, becoming the State Painter under Charles II and James II. William III honoured him with knighthood and Oxford gave him the degree of LLD. He painted many portraits, which were evidently flattering and elegant, for he was made a Baronet by George I and Leopold gave him a patent of nobility.

[53] Sir Anthony Vandyck, a well known Dutch painter who studied under Rubens, resided for a time in Rome and Genoa. On return to Flanders he became so well known, that Cardinal Richelieu invited him to France, but he went to England where Charles I made him a knight. His best work was done in England with historical subjects and portraits. He was interred in St Paul's Cathedral.

[54] Veronese was a celebrated Italian Painter who regarded Titian and Tintoretto as the ultimate painters. He became the leading painter in Venice of the sixteenth century. Like Titian and other painters mentioned, he did not paint at Hampton Court, although portraits of

next room is the Audience Chamber. There are five beautiful paintings by S. Ricci,[57] *Our Savior in the Rich Man's House, Christ Healing the Sick, The Women taken in Adultery, The Women of Faith, The Women of Samoria.* *Ignatius Loyola* by Titian – *Venus and Cupid* by Rubens[58] – the same by Titian, etc. The fifth Chamber is the King's drawing room – George 3rd and the Duke of York reviewing the troops and two painting of Joseph and Potiphan's (?) Wife...

The sixth apartment is King Wm 3rd bedroom in which is placed the State bed of Queen Charlotte. The furniture is a most beautiful specimen embroidered needlework. The ceiling

---

royalty might have been brought to this palace and since then returned to other palaces.

[55] Sir Joshua Reynolds was born in Devonshire in 1723, son of a clergyman who wanted his son to become a doctor. However, the youth's talents prevailed. He studied under a portrait painter by the name of Hudson and later went to Italy for two years of study. After he returned to London, he shortly became a well known portrait painter. First he was president of the Royal Academy, and then he was knighted by the king. His literary ability was recognised by the prominent writers of the day – Johnson, Burke, Goldsmith and Garrick. He is buried at St Paul's Cathedral.

[56] Titian was one of the best known Italian painters from Venice, and was a student of Bellini and Giorgione. He was knighted and given a pension by his king, Charles V. Titian painted history, portraits and landscapes, most of them in Venice and Madrid.

[57] Sebastian Ricci or Rizzi was an Italian painter who worked in Vienna, Paris and for ten years in London. While in England he painted the cupola of Chelsea Hospital – *Ascension.* He left London when Sir James Thornhill, rather than himself, was appointed to paint the dome of St Paul's Cathedral.

[58] Peter Paul Rubens, one of the greatest of the Flemish painters, had studied principally the works of Titian and Veronese in Italy, but had visited Rome, Florence, and other Italian cities before settling in Antwerp. After he became famous he was called to France and Spain and later to England as ambassador from the King of Spain. He became a favourite of Charles I, who made him a knight.

was painted by Verrio and represents Night and Morning – the clock which stands at the head of the bed goes twelve months without winding up. Round the room are the celebrated portraits of Charles 2nd court by Sir Peter Laly,[59] among which the Nell Gwynne[60] – if that portrait is correct she must have been a most beautiful woman, and so indeed were nearly all of them – I never saw a collection of more beautiful women than those portraits exhibited. The seventh chamber is the King's dressing-room. The $ (?) the King's urinating Closet both hung with Pictures by the first master. The 9th and last of the suite is Queen's Mary's Closet – in this room are some fine curious old portraits – Queen Elizabeth when young and when old, Charles II and Francis 23rd when boys, Henry VIII etc.

These rooms all look out upon the gardens and between the windows are large fine mirrors. The doors and lining of them are made of oak highly polished and wrought.[61]

---

[59] Sir Peter Laly originally painted landscapes and historical subjects in the Netherlands, but became an important portrait painter in England. He was noted for his rendering of hands and faces. A favourite of Charles I and Charles II, the latter knighted him. Since the fire, many of these portraits have been removed to other royal palaces or museums. Tapestries cover many walls which were formerly hung with paintings.

[60] Nell Gwynne was a beautiful actress who was a favourite of Charles II. She had started her career as a tavern entertainer.

[61] The curator of the Royal Palaces asked for a copy of the above since little was known of the palace when it was opened to the public by Queen Victoria in 1836.

Dear Mr Reed Ferguson,

I am extremely grateful for the parcel that I received in the post today. It's absolutely marvellous to have a copy of your diary and I will certainly mention it to any publishers here who are interested.

Monday, August 1, 1836 – Went to the Haymarket Theatre[62] to see *The Tragedy of Lori*. Written by Sergeant Talfour, Performed [by] Vanderhoff acted the part of the King Adrastus and Miss Ellen Tree that of Lori. They were the only two reasonably good actors that appeared. Miss Tree certainly possesses much merit, though I think not well calculated for that character. They were both received with boundless applause and loudly called for at the end of the play. Boxes 5 Shillings ($1.15) pit 3 Shillings($.69).

The house is rather smaller than Chestnut St. Theatre[63] and the decorations far inferior. The scenery is very poor. *Make*

I have not yet had time to study it fully but it does look as if it has much useful information in it for us. Your footnotes also seem most illuminating and I am grateful to have the benefit of these as well. Once I have read it and had a chance to show it to my colleagues, I will pass on any relevant comments that they have.

Yours sincerely,

Simon Thurley

[62] The Haymarket Theatre opened in December 1720 and became the Royal Theatre in Haymarket. A second theatre was built in 1821 and became known as the Theatre Royal Haymarket. The theatre has been rebuilt several times, reopening in 1880 and 1905. The only vestige of the theatre JSC would recognise are the six Corinthian Columns forming the portico over the entrance, the same is true of the Drury Lane theatre.

[63] Chestnut Street Theatre, of Philadelphia, Pennsylvania, where JSC went to medical school, is known as 'Old Drury'. It was built on Chestnut west of sixth street in 1793, and was designed by Benjamin Henry Latrobe. It was considered the most elegant and palatial theatre yet constructed in America at the time. However, it burned April 2, 1820, but was rebuilt with William Strickland as the architect. Like the old theatre, there were three horseshoe balconies with burnished gold ornaments of chaste and appropriate designs placed around the

your Wills and *Rural Felicity* two farces were played after *Lori*
the latter is a mutilation of *Rochester*.

Tuesday, August 2nd – Mr. I. Herve, whom I had seen in
Paris last winter called, he resided for a number of years in
different parts of the U.S.as a painter and professor. He is man
of great industry and I should think of considerable talent. He
is about publishing a work on theU.S. He thinks that there are
no men in the English Parliament equal the eloquence to
Webster[64] or Clay[65] and no writer in the English language equal
or to be compared to Channing[66].

Dr Tucker sent me a number of the <u>France Departmentale</u>
containing an article by Dr Baily[67] in which he makes

---

tiers of boxes. The proscenium has a profusion of decorations with
Arabesque devices in green and gold. It opened to the public on
December 22, 1822.

[64]Daniel Webster, a New Hampshire Lawyer, was elected to Congress
in 1813 and to the U.S. Senate in 1828. In 1836, at the time JSC was
in London, he ran unsuccessfully for President.

[65] Henry Clay from Kentucky, was elected to the U.S. Senate in 1809.
He helped negotiate the Treaty of Ghent which ended the War of 1812
with England. He ran for President in 1823, 1832, 1836 and 1844
unsuccessfully.

[66] William Ellery Channing a contemporary of JSC, was a Unitarian
minister noted not only for his preaching, but also for his writing. His
works on John Milton and Napoleon Bonaparte were well recognised
in England.

[67] A quotation from the article by Dr Bailly was published in London
in *The Courier*, Monday Evening, August 15, 1836. Paris, August 16
Extract from the article of Dr Bailly:
'So that he who is afflicted with rupture, is not only condemned for
life to suffered without relaxation the pain and inconvenience produced
by a truss, but he is also exposed to numerous chances of cruel
operation, which proves fatal in at least ten cases out of a hundred.
One must be a physician and an anatomist, to admire how a poor
backwoodsman has been able to imagine an appeal so ingenious and so

favourable mention of the American plan of curing Hernia – calls it *une decouverte admirable et appartenant desormais a la science de*. The article is headed 'Science des masrist'(?) & 'Science des scarces' (?)

I went last night to the English Opera House[68], Wellington St. *The Rose of the Alambra* was Played which is a story of Washington Irving[69] dramatised. Miss Sheriff & Mr Wilson the two principal performers are tolerable singers, but miserable actors, particularly the latter. Mr Hackett the American comedian appeared in the character of Col. Nimrod Wildfire, and elicited great applause. After which *The Farmer's Story* a domestic drama. Stephen Lockwood and Mary his wife, the

---

well adapted to nature the parts upon which it ought to act. This method, so efficacious, gives no pain, and can cause no danger.

'Dr Mott, the Dupuytren of the United States, Professor of Surgery in the University of New York, regards this discovery as 'one of the greatest modern blessings to the human race.'

'Dr Samuel Jackson, Professor in the University of Pennsylvania, and Correspondent of the Institute of France; Granville Sharp Pattison and George McClellan, Professors in the College of Medicine at Philadelphia; William Gibson and William Horner, Professor of Surgery and Anatomy in the University of Pennsylvania, and other celebrated men of America, press forward to proclaim this discovery as an immense service rendered to Humanity.

'It is this method which the Drs Carpenter and Herisson have perfected in France, &c, &c.

'It is this method which Dr Carpenter is now introducing in this city. The cure is effected in from twenty to forty days, without pain, danger or interruption of business. Dr Carpenter can be consulted daily from ten till three – 7 Sacksville Street, Piccadilly.'

[68] The English Opera House or Lyceum Theatre at the corner of Wellington Street, Strand, was built in 1834. It is no longer in existence.

[69] Washington Irving, the American writer, was popular in England where he served as Secretary of the American Legation starting in 1829. He was honoured by the Royal Society of Literature and by Oxford with an LLD.

two principal characters were well supported by Mr Serle and Mrs Fitzwilliam. The story inculcates a good moral – at least a good moral may be extracted from it.

I must not forget to mention Mr Oxberry, who played the rustic the raw country boy. He is an excellent personification of a part English working class.

Thursday, August 4, 1836 – Dine at the Blue Posts[70] Haymarket – pleasant dining-room newspapers – Fried sole, mutton chops & potatoes with a pint of ale – 2s 4d. Called at the Standard office verified the insertion and paid 1.16 pounds ($8.18) for six more insertions, paid John Bull one pound ($4.50) for two insertions.

Went the New Strand Theatre[71] the first entertainment was the Bill Stickers – badly played and contained many allusions which I did not understand. The next was a piece called *Hercules* – the character of Hercules was well supported by W.G. Hammond, the only one worth mentioning. This was followed by a burletta called *P.L. Poet Laureate* or *30 Strand*. The conclusion however, was very amusing, entitled an Operatic Burlesque Burletta, called *Othello*, (according to an act of Parliament). It seems that the theatres of Covent Garden and Drury Lane have a monopoly for playing the legitimate drama, and the other theatres subject themselves to a Penalty by performing them. This Burletta then is a burlesque on the

---

[70] A Blue Post Coffee House existed 1819-1833. It is mentioned in 1838 as 'Blue Posts'. The name came from a method of advertising. A post was erected and painted blue, the name survived the post. None of the places where JSC had dinner are in existence today.

[71] The New Strand Theatre originally opened under a different name in 1803, but it became a chapel for a short time about 1830 before being converted. The New Strand (Subscription) theatre, opened on the 26 January, 1832. The subscription was dropped, but the theatre survived until 1850, reopening several times until 1882, completely rebuilt and enlarged, and it survived until 1905. It was replaced by an Underground station.

42

tragedy of Othello. The Moor is represented by an independent
nigger from Hayti (W. G. Hammond). Iago by a big raw
fisherman from the county of Tipperary. The humour of the
play consisted in the doggerel verses which were said or sung
in the heroical or tender vein as suited the subject – many of
those songs were set to the tune of our finest songs such as
moore(?) & melodies, 'Believe me if all those Endearing young
charms – Come rest in his bosom – ' were song to the most
ridiculous parodies of the imagination. It is a burlesque on the
Italian opera, on the *Tragedy of Othello*, and of our most
favoured songs. It is altogether very ridiculous but one must go
once to such places, but once is always enough for me.

Friday, August 5th 1836 – Received a letter this morning
(via Paris) from Camilla, dated 3rd & 4th July acknowledging a
letter from me dated May 21st and enclosing a draft for
$100.00. On the 8th of June I wrote from Paris to let her know
of my change of plans – I arrived in London the 13th and did
not write to her, I believe until the lst of July.

Went the Queen's Theatre,[72] Tottenham St. Tottenham
Court, Tottenham Road, where there is a French company
performing, *Malade Imaginair. Chez la Duchess du Barry dans
le temps de Louis XV Singing by Madam Grise, Tambusini
Lablache & Rulini.* Dancing by Mademoiselle Grise etc. The
company is not strong nor effective, Laporte who sustained the
principle character was the principal attraction. Grise & the

---

[72] Queen's Theatre was created in 1829 from a house, tennis court and
billiard room. It was a private subscription theatre. By 1833, under a
new regime, it became the Queen Theatre, Tottenham Street.
Between 1833-1835 the name was changed several times and finally
Lord Chamberlain closed the theatre, but opened it again as Cooke's
Circus and theatre. Later it became a waxworks with a increasingly
poor reputation. In the twentieth century a restaurant, casino and
bowling alley have replaced the theatre.

other celebrated singers merely gave one piece of music each. The dancing was admirable.

Sat alongside an English lady who has traveled a good deal – was very curious about America. A fat woman sat before me who asked me what principal towns were nearest Philadelphia and was quite surprised to hear that it was a large city.

Saturday, August 6 1836 – Read, *Mrs Arymitage or Female Domination*. Dined at an Oyster house in the Haymarket – a dish of stewed oysters and a crab, bread and butter. 2s 6d.

The crab crawled about my stomach all night, and I dreamed a dream – an old hag wanted to give me poison to drink, to which I objected, whereas she was highly displeased, etc. I have forsworn crabs – I may live to be crabbed but never to eat crab.

Sunday, August 7, 1836 – Dined at Verry's[73] *Potage Julienne-Fricandeau a la sauce tomato – despetits pories a le Francaise* 2s 6d ($.58). Took a long walk from there to Hyde Park over the serpentine[74] & along its banks, etc.

Tuesday, August 9 1816 – Bought at No.60 St Paul's Church yard,[75] the following articles, & sent them to Camilla

---

[73] Verry's restaurant, 233 Regent Street, was one of the leading Victorian restaurants. Included in the celebrity patrons were the Prince of Wales, Disraeli and Charles Dickens. The restaurant is no longer in existence.

[74] The Serpentine was a lake in Kensington Gardens and Hyde Park used frequently in summer for bathing and in winter for ice skating. A somewhat smaller lake still exists.

[75] St Paul's, originally as designed by Indigo Jones, was intended to have been surrounded by a colonnade; but only the north and a part of the east side were completed. The west side was occupied by fruit and vegetable markets which were completed in 1829-30. There were wholesale establishments on the south side of St Paul's Churchyard, where one could shop if a letter of introduction was secured.

by her father: Four Capes – 2 10 pounds ($11.30), two muslin dresses 2.18 pounds ($13.00), six yards sateen for the children 14 S.3 ($3.25) = 6.2.3 pounds (total). Gave Mr Sanderson fifty three pounds ($103.50) and paid his tailor's bill which amounted to – (no amount).

We went in the evening to an oyster house in the Haymarket and had some scallope and stewed oysters and a pint of port wine – cost five shillings ($1.15). Wrote to John Sanderson... by his father. Wrote to Camilla but forgot to give him the letter.

Wednesday, August 10, 1836 – Mr Sanderson[76] left London today in the stage for Portsmouth with the Smith family, they visit the Isle of Wight on the way to Le Havre. Went to Mr Smith's and saw them off – met there M. Seurrier and another Monsieur. Bought Camilla an *L'Italie par Mme De Stall* for 7s ($1.61) an old English Bible printed in 1619 for 18s ($4.14).

Thursday, August 11 1836 – Read *The Pirates and Cutters* by Capt. Marvatt.[77] Visited the gallery of Mechanical Arts Loreat(?) arcade where are congregated many useful inventions, machines, models of ships, steamboats, a steam engine, Hydro – oxygen, Microscope etc.

Went to the Haymarket Theatre at nine o'clock, paid half price. *The Young Queen* or *Christine of Sweden, The Second Sight* and *My Husband's Ghost* were all performed after nine

---

[76] Mr Sanderson, JSC's father-in-law, had been in France for over a year. The young doctor had been with him in Paris for six months.

[77] Frederick Marryat (1792-1848) a naval officer – Commander at age twenty-three – and novelist: he published his first novel at thirty-seven. After resigning from the Navy, he published *The King's Own* and started editing *Metropolitan Magazine*. He went to America in 1837 for two years. During his writing career, he wrote ten novels and many short stories. The robust humour of his books helped the popularity.

o'clock. The Theatre did not close until after one. Sinclair sang some good songs and Miss Taylor acted, Mrs Musket very well. Miss Ellen Nees' Queen had rather too much of affected majesty in it to be natural or agreeable.

Friday, August 12th – Received a letter from Camilla dated P.V. [Pottsville] July 11th via Paris – has recd. no letters from me since May 21st which she acknowledged in her last letter.

Translated Mr Erving's letter to the Editor of the Temps (?), and some extracts from Dr Bailly's article and paid 25 S to *The Courier* for its insertion.

Dined in an oyster house on two dozen oysters, bread and butter and a pint of porter. price 2s ($.46). The oysters called natives are considered the best, but they are very small and have a slight coppery taste.

Accosted by a man in the street, who asked me if I wanted to buy a box of good Segars or other articles in his line. It appears that he is an agent for the smugglers.

Saturday, Aug 13th – Took my letter to Camilla to the N.&SA. Coffee House[78] where I dined – called on Mr Eccles who invited me to dine with him on Monday. Took Coffee with him and afterwards called on Dr Crucifix, Wellington St. who was not home. Went with him to the Strand theatre where was performed the Bill Sticker, *Hercules* the King of Clubs and the Burletta of *Othello* – went after that was over to the Rainbow House[79] near the Temple Bar, took some oysters &

---

[78] The N&SA Coffee House was North and South American Coffee House on Threadneedle Street, located near the present day Bank of England and the Royal Exchange. The Post Office Directory of 1839 lists James Davis as proprietor.

[79] A frequently used name in the nineteenth century, which cannot be identified.

stout. The house has the reputation of keeping the best stout in London.

Sunday, Aug. 14th – Went to Westminster Abbey & listened to the music & wandered about among the tombs of the mighty dead. As you enter the door at Poet's Corner, the first bust is that of Ben Jonson! with this pithy line underneath – 'O rare Ben Jonson'.[80] Along side is placed Milton – Dryden and over the door of the Western and Goldsmith.

Dined at Verry's, walking around Park Crescent & Regent Park. I followed a stream of people & entered a large church in New Road. It is a very large building with two tiers of Galleries, one over the other – evangelical a low church I think.

Monday, August 15th – Read Capt. Maryatt's New Novel – *"Rattlin the Reefer"*. It is by no means equal to his former productions. Dined with Mr Eccles – met Dr Myers, served in the Army in Spain during the last war. Mr Barrow an elderly gentleman and Messrs. Brown. Mr Geo Eccles called in after dinner and invited me to dine with him on Sunday next. Mr Bickers send for two dozen pamphlets – sent him twenty-six.

Wednesday, August 17 – Commenced taking *The Times* newspaper. It is to be brought to me every morning for one shilling ($.23) per week – to keep it an hour and a half or two hours. Trussed the Captain Wynne who gave me his agent's name – to pay 20 pounds ($90.00) when cured. He is on Half pay – has served under Wellington in Spain.

Thursday, 18th August – Dined at Short & Shand Hotel, opposite Somerset House which was recommended to me by Capt Wynne. Soup, fish and hot Joint of the best quality price 1 S 6 p ($.35) – silver forks excellent room & good company.

---

[80] The phrase "O Rare Ben Jonson" also is painted on a stone near the floor on the north aisle not far from the entrance to the Abbey.

It is the best & cheapest place to dine at that I have found. Went to Exeter Hall to hear the abolitionist Geo Thompson[81] lecture. He possesses some power of eloquence and more enthusiasm. His lecture was a tirade on the evils of slavery – the duty & necessity of immediate and entire abolition of slavery with some exaggerated account of the state of abolition societies in the US. After he sat down the secretary of the meeting made a speech on the causes of the present war in Texas.[82]

Friday, August 19th, 1836 – My cousin Samuel T. Jones of Manchester, called yesterday while I was out, left his card. This evening I called to see him at the London Coffee House and we went to the Colliseum together.[83] It is a vast building containing a theatre, Hall of Mirrors – a large circular room

---

[81] George Thompson (1804-1878). An Anti-Slavery advocate. Starting in 1833 a series of lectures lead to the formation of the 'Edinburgh Society for the Abolition of Slavery Throughout the World'. In 1834 he went to the United States and engaged with Americans in the Anti-Slavery Movement which in time founded over three hundred branch associations. He was denounced by General Jackson in a Presidential message. As his life was endangered, he escaped to a ship bound for England, his return was received with enthusiasm. In 1851 he returned to the States and for a third time during the Civil War. During this visit he was given a public reception by the House of Representatives in the presence of President Lincoln.

[82] In 1836, more than two hundred Texans fought and won independence from Mexico at the Battle of the Alamo and San Jacinto... The defenders, including Davy Crockett and Jim Bowie, died in the long siege against four thousand Mexicans under General Santa Anna, but the Independence of Texas was shortly declared with Sam Houston as president.

[83] No information could be found regarding Samuel T. Jones, a cousin, or the London Coffee House. The Coliseum was located in the south-eastern corner of Regent's Park and was closed in the 1870s.

devoted to the fine arts, a conservatory – Alpine Scenery, surfs cottages, grotto & caves etc.

In the theatre we had some singing, a ballet, and the wonderful performances of the Bedouin Arabs, consisting of feats of agility & strength that I have never seen equalled.

Herr Weiner's Zoological concert was very curious. He imitates the noise of various animals in the most perfect manner. The singing of birds, the barking of dogs – the caterwauling of cats etc. He is a blind German. Child's dissolvent views are also well worth seeing. The Hall of Mirrors is very beautiful – as the name imparts. It is filled with them. The pillars which are octagon are covered them & the angles concealed by gilt strips. The ceiling is painted with arabesque.

Sunday, 21 August – Went to church All Saints,[84] I think it is called, in Regents Street, well attended, good sermon. Called at the London Coffee House on my way to Geo. Eccles' – for some letters. Dined at Mr. G. Eccles[85] – Met Monsieur Cheville a French teacher and Mr Russel – examined two of Mr E's children who are affected slight umbilical ruptures. The mother has also the same complaint. Promised to attend to them.

Monday, August 22 – This is the King's Birth Day,[86] but I see no signs of rejoicing. No *fete du Roi* as in Paris, but people

---

[84] All Soul's Church is located on Langham Place, an extension of Regent Street.

[85] George Eccles was a printer and lithographer (101 French Church Street). He probably printed the brochures that JSC was distributing. Wm. Eccles (12 Union or Old Broad Street) was a surgeon.

[86] When JSC was in London, William IV was king of England. He had been in the Royal Navy since the age of fifteen, retiring aged forty. Upon the death of his brother George IV in 1830, he became king and ruled until 1837, when at his death Princess Victoria became Queen.

attend their business as if His Gracious Majesty has never been born, or as if he was a mere man of straw, set on the British Throne to cover the acts of his ministers. It is said that it will be celebrated at Windsor, the Royal residence. Called at the Times office and paid 1 pound 16s ($8.18) for six insertions of my advertisement to be put in daily.

Wednesday, August 24 – I am very much amused with some of my patients. I like to study their characters & observe their peculiarities – Capt... is a half-pay officer having been battered about in the Peninsular War under Wellington. Ruined his constitution by lues[87] Mercury and exposure – afflicted with two hernias etc. He has nothing to do but spend his time & his seven Shillings ($1.61) a day in the best way he can. He uses the term "the consequence was" in all manner of ways.

Speaking of the poor, a fellow brought before the turtle fed alderman, on a charge of stealing a piece of bread. The consequence was the poor man said he was so hungry he couldn't help it. Damn your eyes, said the alderman, I'd give a thousand pounds for your appetite – & dismissed him with five shillings ($1.15). These aldermen," said the Capt, "they make money in such a dam obstinate kind of a way that the consequence is they have no appetite!

Saturday, 27th August – Yesterday went to the Lancet office bought ten books containing Broussais (?) lectures on Phrenology[88] and directed the work to be sent me every week.

Bought of Mr... Parkin, No. 440 Shand, a razor which he warrants, price 7 S ($.1.61) & a pot of shaving soap price 2s 6d (about $.50).

---

[87] Syphilis.

[88] Phrenology is a study of the conformation of the skull based on the belief that it is indicative of mental faculties and character.

Saturday, 28th – Finished reading Madame de Stael's[89] *Corinne*, admirable work – what a charm she throws over the classic soil of Italy! How beautiful are her descriptions! Called on Mr Eccles, surgeon – went to a dissenting chapel. Presbyterian, I believe. Spent the evening at home reading the Bible. There are many parts of this book which in any other form or shape would be considered highly improper and injurious to the morals of its readers.

Tuesday, August 30th – Bought two woollen shirts (knit), for a crown[90] apiece – Holland linen for thirty shillings ($6.90) & a cashmere for sixteen do (?).

Wednesday, August 31st – Read *Lybney Hall* by Thos Hood[91] author of the Comic Annual. As a whole it is interesting & displays considerable power of description &

---

[89] Anne Germaine de Stael, a French author and daughter of Necker, Minister of Finance under Louis XVI. She was well-educated and started writing plays as well as short stories. She first attracted attention by *Letters upon the Writings and Character of Rousseau* (1778). She was married the much older Swedish ambassador to France, and so during the Revolution was permitted to remain. Her sympathies changed from supporting the revolutionaries to defending Marie Antoinette. She was forced to flee until the establishment of the Directory. Under Bonaparte, she went to Switzerland and Italy, described in her novels *Delphone* and *Corinne*. Later, writing about Germany and visiting England, she was warned by Napoleon's Minister of Police to stay out of France. One of her major works was *Ten Years of Exile*, a denunciation of Napoleon and later, *Considerations sur la Revolution Francaise*. She was a very remarkable woman in a very difficult time in France.

[90] A Crown is a silver United Kingdom coin with a value of five shillings or about seventy cents in American Money.

[91] Thomas Hood 1799-1845, poet humorist editor. Assistant Editor *London Magazine* 1821. In 1830 started *Comic Annual* later became a playwright.

definition of character – but there is too much hard straining after the witty & the ludicrous – to much of the comic Almanac.

"Life itself was new,
And the heart promises what the fancy drew"

But when I mingled with the chafing 'tides of human existence' in Cheapside[92], my heart sunk within me, I felt, as it were annihilated – lost, like a drop of water in the ocean – overwhelmed in the tumultuous stream of living beings that flowed around me.   There are few who have not felt this on first mixing with the crowd in the streets of London.

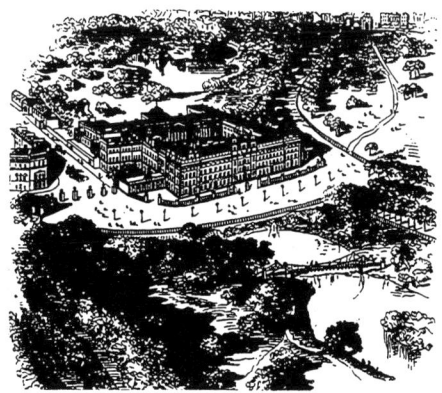

Buckingham Palace, and the West End of St James's Park

Friday, September 2nd – visited Buckingham Palace[93] with Dr Carroll. It is finished and furnished, but the King does not

---

[92] Cheapside in JSC's day, one of the oldest and most famous streets of London, near St Paul's Cathedral.
[93] Buckingham Palace is the residence of the King and Queen of England. Formerly known as Buckingham House, it was built in 1703 by the Duke of Buckingham and later bought by King George III in 1762 for twenty-one thousand pounds. Altered by Nash for George IV, in 1825 the name was changed to Buckingham Palace, however, it was seldom used as the official residence (the King preferred St James

like it. So lives in the old barn called St James[94], and his nation has spent some millions for nothing.

We entered from St James Park, the entrance Hall ascending a few steps into the Hall of Sculpture, running the whole length of the main building – The private dining-room contains a painting of the opening of new London Bridge, Malta & the Quarantine Harbour of Malta. The ante room to the library. The library – Council Room – Kings Private Library are all on the ground floor. Ascending the grand staircase we entered the salon, richly carpeted containing two rich and curiously inlaid cabinets ornamented with precious stones. The throne room occupies the last end of the first floor in front. The middle of this floor is intended for a picture gallery and is lighted from above. It contains only three or four statues by Chantry.[95] The back part of this floor contains the drawing-rooms, very richly furnished. In the bow room is a beautiful table inlaid with cameo's of ancient heroes & said to have been presented to George IV by Napoleon. The Queen's bedroom – sleeping room – rooms for the Ladies in Waiting & etc. are in the East wing – servants apartments in the west.

Palace) until Queen Victoria came to the throne in 1837 and added the East Wing.

[94] St James's Palace was built by Henry VIII, an 'inelegant brick structure' in 1530. This palace was used only occasionally by Queen Victoria when she ascended the throne. The Chapel Royal (the ceiling probably designed by Holbein in 1530) was the scene of many royal weddings, including that of Prince Albert and Queen Victoria 1840, and King George and Queen Mary (1893). Today it is the home of the Queen Mother.

[95] Sir Francis Legatt Chantrey (1781-1841) was first a painter and later a well known sculptor, primarily of portrait busts. A list of his work would catalogue the names of most of the distinguished men of his time, including Sir Walter Scott, Wordsworth, James Watt and many others. He was very popular when JSC was in London. His works are in all the major British museums, palaces and public buildings.

Sunday, September 4th, 1836
Tuesday, September 6th

[Diary for Sunday September 4 and Tuesday September 6 was medical.]

Thursday, September 8th – Recd. a letter from Camilla, dated August 4th. & one from Dr Tucker [French partner].

Note to Camilla took it to the N&SAC house. Go the 10th. This is the anniversary of King's Coronation – a few flags hung out, is the only demonstration of honour that I have observed.

Read *The King's Own* by Capt. Marryat. Like the man who read the Dictionary and being asked how he liked it said, pretty well, only it don't end well – I liked the book generally, but it ends badly. Shipwreck, murders, dreadful accidents, poisoning, suicide etc. The last chapter is a conglomeration of horrors.

Friday, September 9th – News from New York by the Packet ship Oxford up to the 17th arrived in Liverpool on Wednesday.

Sunday, September 11th – Went with Dr C. to visit Kensington Gardens, or rather Park for there are no gardens, but immediately around the Palace. It is a most noble Park, full of magnificent trees and covered with a rich and smooth and green a turf as I have ever beheld. Seats are placed about under the trees and occasionally a little round building in case of rain. The Duchess of Kent the Princess Victoria reside at this palace.

Monday, September 12th – Recd. a letter from Camilla dated August 11 and from its being directed to Sacksville St. She must have recd. my letter of July 1.

Thursday, 15 September – Recd. a note from Mr G. Eccles, stating that the two hundred and fifty copies of my pamphlet had been disposed of, and wishing to know if he should print a few more until I could prepare matter for the second edition.

Rode up to St. John's wood near Paddington[96] and dined at the Yorkshire...(?) Mr. Myers invited me to dine with him tomorrow 7 New Church St.

Friday, September 16 – Dined at Mr Myers, surgeon, with W. Eccles and a Mr Garect; the latter lived for several years in Frankfort near Phila. Flax spinner (?) Myers served as surgeon in Spain and Portugal during the Peninsular War. He is now a general practitioner i.e. an apothecary surgeon and accoucheur.[97]

Sunday 18th – I went into the City today to hear a Mr Fox[98] who has the reputation of considerable eloquence. The service commenced with a prayer and a hymn – the subject of his discourse was poetry. His religion appears to be benevolence – the cultivation of reason his chief object.

Monday, September 19th – City of London School – founded by John Carpenter.[99] Thos Brewster has compiled a

---

[96] Paddington was a delightful little rustic village in the eighteenth to nineteenth century.

[97] Obstetrician.

[98] William Johnson Fox (1786-1864), Preacher, politician, writer. He became popular as a liberal speaker and later was elected to Parliament. Fox was a prolific writer on liberal subjects as well as religion.

[99] John Carpenter (1370?-1441?) not a relative, Town Clerk of London for a number of years, frequently addressed letters to Henry V. During his term he compiled the laws, customs, privileges and usages of the city extracting them from the archives. His writing and extract of laws were printed as *Liber Albus* from the manuscript in 1859. He became a Member of Parliament in 1436, was later given

memoir of him. In the reign of Henry VI a certain estate were devised to the corporation by Carpenter who was town clerk for the purpose of educating, clothing, & maintaining four poor boys. By increased value of the land, a school which is now in progress of erection, on the site of honey lane market, is endowed with the annual sum of 900 pounds! Carpenter is well known in civic history. He was not only skilled in that knowledge of the laws of the city which as town Clerk it was his duty to possess, but he deserves to be ranked amongst the patrons of the fine arts since it was at his expense and under his patronage, that the famous "Macabre" or Dance of Death was painted in St Paul's cloister. The opinion of his moral worth and the high estimation in which he was held by his fellow citizens is shown by the fact of his having been appointed executor to the celebrated Whyttington, as well as two other citizens, the execution of which offices involved the performance of various charitable trusts, and a consequence heavy responsibility. In his office he has immortalised his name by the compilation of a large volume on matters relating to the city. It is still deemed of the highest authority & has been used with such effect that its original name, (Liber Albus) has given way to another indication of its state from constant use. (Liber Niger)   *The Times*, 19 September

Tuesday, 20 September 1836 – Yesterday I got into conversation with a Scotchman from the town of Edinburgh. I like the Scotch they have a vast fund of dry humour and of good sense, not to be found among the beer drinking English. He took me to be a Glasgow man from my accent. Read a new

---

honorary knighthood. During his many years of service, he was well reimbursed and when he died he left the money to establish a new school and university as well as a number of scholarships. The school was called City of London School

work by Alan Cunningham[100] called, *Lord Boldan* – the writer is a true Scotsman there are a great many good things in his work – but are many parts of the story very improbable and a good deal of superstition.

Wednesday, 21 September – Recd. a letter from James Brown, M.D. Professor of Midwifering at Andersonian University, Glasgow which I answered. Wrote a note to Mr Rifnor in I suspect not very good French.

Had a fire made for the first time this season, though it has been quite cold enough the whole of this month for a fire to be acceptable.

From examination of commissioners made in Ireland, there appears to be an incredible amount of misery and destitution. Starvation stalks through their land – not more than three persons out of two hundred among the labourmen can afford to mix a little buttermilk amongst their potatoes.

Whole families live for weeks on one meal a day – that composed of [?] cabbage boiled with a little meal.

---

[100] Allan Cunningham 1784-1842, was a Scottish poet and biographer from Dumfriesshire, where Robert Burns was buried. Cunningham walked in the funeral procession of Robert Burns. His books were novels, biographies (Burns) dramas and critical historical notes. He was highly respected by Sir Walter Scott, Hogg (another Scottish poet) and Chantrey.

Random Recollections of the House of Lord's Tory Party.

Duke of Cumberland[101] – His Royal Highness wearing large whiskers & mustachios of a milky white appearance – no speaker – a man of no talent – not the remotest pretensions to intellect of any kind-ignorant of the plainest rules of composition.

Duke of Wellington[102] – The most distinguished man of the Present day, as a General, not as a statesman. Great moral courage – indifferent to popularity. General information neither varied or profound. Were his diction & manner good His Grace would rank high as a speaker, but both are bad – bad voice, great energy of manner. Age 67, hair greyish, face pale & drawn-eye keen of countenance. Indication of energy & determination – rather above middle size-slender and very

---

[101] Duke of Cumberland was Ernest Augustus (1771-1851) who had a great influence on the King. He was always a mischief maker. Wellington made a formal complaint about him.

[102] Duke of Wellington was born Arthur Wellesley, third son of the Earl of Mornington (1767-1852). Biographer Elizabeth Longford says he was born in the same year as Napoleon. He attended Eton and Royal Academy of Equitation in France; at twenty-seven he went to India where he became a scholar and soldier, returning as Knight of Bath, a Major General. He took command of the Allied armies in the Peninsular War which ended with the defeat of Napoleon and his exile to Elba. After Napoleon's escape, Wellington lead the British and Dutch-Belgium armies to the defeat of Napoleon at Waterloo. Wellington's military career ended with this battle and many have said that it was just his beginning as the 'Pillar of State'. He became Prime Minister of a country needing reforms. He considered himself a servant of the King and the people. Queen Victoria did not appreciate him at first, but later needed his help. In 1841 he wrote, "The truth is that all I desire is to be as useful as possible to the Queen's service – to do anything, go anywhere, and hold any office, or no office, as may be thought most desirable." He was five feet nine inches tall, muscular with penetrating grey eyes. His chief characteristic was his manliness and his public spirit. He is buried beside fellow-hero, Nelson, in St Paul's Cathedral.

erect. Partial to blue coat, light vest & trousers – not well made.

Duke of Gordon[103] – ultra Tory – never speaks in the House, detests liberal principles – great promotion of Orangeism. Age 66. Tall & handsome in person – hair grey features handsome, face oval – complexion ruddy – appearance commanding & dignified.

Duke of Newcastle[104] – An ultra Tory active in politics – very tall, very stout & unwieldy in his physical conformation – features large strongly marked – age 50.

Duke of Buckingham[105] – Immense, pot-bellied, jolly and fond of quizzing – bad speaker, both in manner & matter – very few ideas but fond of quoting Shakespeare, and palming them off for his own. Age 60.

Duke of Northumberland[106] – never speaks in the House – has a revenue of pounds 250,000 per annum – has as much as

---

[103] The Duke of Gordon (1770-1836) as Marquis of Huntley served with the Guards in Flanders, raised Gordon Highlanders (1795-1799), He became a Lt General 1808, was badly wounded 1819 and later became General, succeeding to the Dukedom in 1827.

[104] Duke of Newcastle – Henry Pelham Fieness Pelham (1785-1851) became the 4th Duke of Newcastle. He studied at Oxford. In 1834 he became a Lord of the Treasury, the first of many government duties he performed. In 1859 he was again appointed secretary for the Colonies, and in 1860 he accompanied the Prince of Wales in his travels in Canada and in the United States where he was held in "great esteem".

[105] Richard Temple Nugent Brydges Chandos Grenville (1776-1839) was the first Duke of Buckingham. He graduated from Oxford and was elevated to Duke by George IV 1822. He lived very extravagantly, with large expenditures for art, literature and entertaining. He went abroad in private yacht for two years (account of travels published in 1862, 3 volumes). Throughout his life he devoted his money, talent and time to collecting.

[106] The Duke of Northumberland was born Hugh Percy III (1785-1847), and was a descendant of one of the most distinguished families

the King – lately <u>Lord Lieutenant of Ireland</u> – rather tall – slender – sandy complexion – suffers from ill health. Appearance & manners gentlemanly without any of the haughtiness of the aristocrat. Age 51.

<u>Duke of Buccleucch</u>[107] – Annual income 250,000 pounds. A Scotchman – speaks but seldom, not the slightest animation in his manners, or energy in his actions. Has given no indication of talent – good looking features, small and regular and wears an expression of mildness approaching to simplicity. Complexion fair, hair sandy – middle height & handsomely made age 30 one of the youngest peers in the house.

Marquises, Tory –

<u>Marquis of Londonderry</u>[108] a most zealous ultra Tory – twice mobbed and narrowly escaped with his life-injuries. He has impudent zeal, his great success is want of Judgement but he is strictly honest and straight forward. He will neither compromise or abandon his principles – neither will he conceal or disguise them. He is a man of honour as well as honesty, but he has no talent, miserable speaker praises Don, Miguel

---

of England. March 1807 brought forward a bill for the abolition of slavery in the colonies; the bill did not pass through Parliament. In 1817 he succeeded his father as the Duke of Northumberland. He was a moderate Tory. He accepted Wellington's offer in 1829 to be Viceroy of Ireland, but asked to be relieved after twelve to eighteen months. He supported the Catholic Association. Later he became a governor of King's College and a trustee of the British Museum, as well as Vice President for the Society of Arts. He has been called a prodigious bore with no political opinions.

[107] Duke of Buccleuch (Buccleucch) 7th Duke of Queensberry (1806-1884). Honorary LLD Cambridge 1842, Edinburgh 1874, Chancellor Glasgow University 1877.

[108] Marquis of Londonderry – Charles Wilson Stewart, had a military career. He served in St Petersburg Embassy 1835. He was also the pole bearer at Wellington's funeral. He published a narrative of Peninsular Campaign 1813-1814.

Don Carlos & their governments – thinks them amiable and... calls them Poles rebels. He is a handsome man above the middle height and well formed complexion rather florid-hair brown features regular and his countenance has a pleasant expression. Age58.

Marquis of Wellesley[109] – great personal resemblance to his relative the Duke of Wellington, but is rather stouter – common height complexion fair and hair of a light colour. His appearance never fails to command veneration. He is a man of some talent but very defection in judgement seldom speaks hasty temper – fluent speaker – few ideas. Age 76. His constitution must have suffered from the fatigue of a long active service, in different parts of the world.

Marquis of Salisbury takes a prominent participation in the proceedings of the House – bad speaker but is brief.

Earls, Tory -
Lord Eldon[110] – Speaker of the House of Lords & 'Keeper of the King's conscience' – Toryism is part and parcel of his existence. After the passage of the Reform Bill he explained "Now the son of England's glory is forever set". He looks on this country... [?] as lost beyond all hope of recovery. A greater stickler for ancient usages & ancient institutions never

---

[109] Marquis de Wellesley – Richard Colley Wellesley (1760-1842), educated at Eton (Latin and Greek) and studied at Christ Church, Oxford until father's death 1781. He was made Governor General of India 1797. His *Indian Despatches* were published in 1836. He was ambassador to Spain for a short time, then Lord Lieutenant of Ireland and later Secretary of State. He was one of the original St Patrick Knights, and a brother of Duke of Wellington. His most important service was the suppression by law of the secret societies – both Protestant and Catholic. See footnote 212

[110] Eldon, John Scott attended Oxford and took a Master of Arts degree(1773). He first served in the House of Lords in 1799 as Baron Eldon. In 1821 he was created Viscount Encombe and Earl of Eldon. He served as a Trustee of the British Museum.

lived. In his view time hallowed everything – (age eighty-five). Not an orator a man of great integrity. He is tall & well formed – remarkable for his venerable appearance – face full – fair complexion – features large – great projection of the eyebrows, giving the eyes a sunken appearance – forehead well developed.

Earl of Wicklow[111] – May be regarded as the leader of the opposition, on all matters relating to Ireland – fair talent – clever in debate – great deal of self esteem – usual height – stout & compact, complexion fair, hair red features regular-face round & pleasing. Age 48.

Earl of Limerick[112] – age 78. One of the most violent Tories in the House, not a man of much talent.

Earl of Winchilsea[113] – chiefly distinguished for his warm attachment to the established church – he's tall & stout complexion dark & has black features, small and regular age 45.

Lord Roden[114] – another champion of the church – his intellectual powers like those of the Earl of Winchilsea, are below mediocrity – hates the Roman Catholics. He is one of the tallest and stoutest men in the House – good looking – dark complexion. Age 48.

Earl of Aberdeen[115] – Ultra Tory – formerly Secretary of Foreign Affairs – has written work on the Antiquities of Athens

---

[111] William Forward 4th (1788) was the Earl of Wicklow.

[112] Edmund Henry Pery, Earl of Limerick and 2nd Baron Glenworth. He was attached to the Protestant Ascendancy party.

[113] George William Finch-Hatton, 5th Earl of Nottingham and 9th Earl of Winchilsea. A violent opponent of Catholic relief, he fought a duel with Wellington in 1829. He was a frequent speaker against liberal measures.

[114] Robert Jocelyn, 3rd Earl of Roden, was a Grand Master of the Orange Society. He was created a British Peer in 1821.

[115] George Hamilton Gordon, Earl of Aberdeen, earned a Masters degree from St John's College, Cambridge in 1804. He founded the Altherian Society; became Ambassador to Vienna 1813; Chancellor of

– dresses with much carelessness – about the middle height dark complexion – a man of taste and intelligence.

Earl of Haddington[116] formerly Lord Lieutenant of Ireland – a man of respected talents – at 46.

Earl of Harrowly[117] – at 74 – President of the Council in the Ministry of Lord Liverpool for many years. Much shrewdness not one of the most Ultra Tories.

Earl of Mansfield at 60 – hair quite grey, rather above the ordinary height and well proportioned good speaker always makes set speeches.

Tory Baron –

Lord Wynford[118] as a lawyer he earned for himself a high reputation – his mind is deficient in vigour – considerable moral courage excellent private character.

Lord Lyndhurst[119] – the ablest man with the exception of Lord Brougham in the House of Lords. As a judge, he is

---

Duchy of Lancaster under Wellington's cabinet; foreign secretary 1828-30; and Secretary of War and Colonies under Lord Peel 1834-5. He is credited with preventing a schism in the Scottish church by Non-Intrusion Act of 1843; later as foreign secretary, he improved the relationship with America by the Oregon Treaty of 1846.

[116] Thomas Hamilton, 9th Earl of Haddington, was educated at Edinburgh and Christ Church, Oxford MA 1815. He was Indian Commissioner; succeeding to the Scottish peerage in 1828. He was Lord Lieutenant of Ireland 1834-35; First Lord of the Admiralty 1840-46; and Lord Privy Seal 1846.

[117] Dudley Ryder, Earl of Harrowly, an MA from St Johns College 1782. He served as Lord of Admiralty 1827-28, and Prime Minister of Liverpool for a number of years. He supported the Reform Bill.

[118] William Draper Best, Tory Baron – Lord Wynford, Deputy speaker House of Lords, was raised to the Peerage in 1829.

[119] Lord Lyndhurst, at about two years of age, was taken by his father to England. He graduated from Trinity College and later studied Law. Early in his career he became well known as an attorney during an important treason trial. Having been given the title of Lord, he

perhaps, surpassed by no one who ever sat on the Bench – few have even equalled him. Formerly Mr. John Singleton Copley – elected to the House of Commons in 1821 by the influence of Lord Liverpool – formerly entertained liberal opinions. Some say he was a red hot republican, this he denies. He is a native of America – his father was a portrait painter. In 1813 he was made sergeant at Law. In 1818 Chief Justice of Chester – in 1819 Solicitor General and a few months afterwards had to appear for government in the prosecution against Queen Caroline – Created Attorney General in 1824 – in 1826 he succeeded Lord Gifford as Master of the Rolls. 1827 he was raised to the highest elevation a subject can attain he was appointed Lord Chancellor, one of the most ingenious Sophist that ever belonged to either House of Parliament – his manner is most insinuating has the most perfect coolness & self possession – cannot be said to be an eloquent speaker – his style is however clear...[?] & simple in no ordinary degree – Addisonian – he is tall and well-made forehead high and well-made mouth of character, nose aquiline, complexion dark –64 years wears a wig.

Lord Ellenborough[120] – Quantity of hair carefully curled – tall and well made, age forty-six, correct speaker but cold.

Lord Ashburton[121] – formerly Alexander Baring considerable talent but inconsistent *The Times* used to call him

---

served in the Upper House until 1846. Even at the age of eighty he delivered remarkable speeches relating to the war with Russia, on Cambridge University reform, life peerages, and the defences of the country.

[120] Edward Law, first Earl of Ellenborough, in 1818 succeeded to the peerage as second baron. In 1828 he was made President of the Board of Control under the administration of Wellington and Sir Robert Peel. In 1842 he was made Governor-General of India, and after returning was made First Lord of the Admiralty. He continued serving in several important capacities for the next decade.

[121] Lord Ashburton, the second son of Sir Francis Baring Bart, was a London merchant of considerable wealth. Upon the death of his father

the representative of his breeches' pocket. Speaks one way and votes another – excels in mystifying his subjects. He is not a firm speaker – his forehead has more of breadth than height – age 56.

Lord Abinger[122] – formerly Sir James Scarlet – a man of considerable acquired talents he realises, in some measure, our ideas Falstaff at 58.

Lord Kenyon is not a man of vigorousness or comprehensive mind. Great supporter of Orangeism. He is an indifferent speaker. At fifty-seven, complexion florid – nose large and aquiline features regular and pleasing, but by no means intellectual.

Press who have seats in the cabinet.

Lord Melbourne[123] – formerly the Hon. William Lamb and then a Tory – he cannot be said to be a man of superior talent – great common sense of considerable reading great moral courage at 57.

Lord Holland[124] – Nephew of Charles James Fox – decided liberal – he is a good speaker & a man of considerable literary attainment at 63.

---

he became head of the firm of Baring Brothers & Co and was shortly elected to Parliament. In 1834 he became a member of Sir Robert Peel's cabinet as President of the Board of Trade and Master of the Mint. In 1841 he went to America and helped settle the Oregon boundary question, 'The Ashburton Treaty'.

[122] The title comes from Abinger, in Surrey.

[123] Lord Melbourne entered the House of Commons in 1805 as a Whig. He was appointed Secretary of State for Ireland, a post he filled with distinguished success. In 1828 he moved to the House of Lords and was a member of Earl Grey's cabinet. In 1834 he became First Lord of the Treasury and head of the Whig party. He was not particularly talented, but his conciliatory manner secured him friends and positions.

[124] Lord Holland was the 3rd Lord and like his father a champion of public liberty. He denounced the war against Napoleon. Published

Marquis of Lansdowne[125] – formerly Lord Petty. When young, great expectations were formed of him – great fluency but more showy than solid. He has no pretensions to vigour or originality of mind. Excels in defiance of measure – not remarkably liberal in his opinions – always cool & collected, but has no energy or decision of character at fifty-seven a striking figure.

Lord Duncanon[126] – Lord Glenleg and Lord Minto are the other members of the Cabinet in the upper House.

Liberal Party, Dukes -

Duke of Sussex[127] – sometimes called 'The popular member of the Royal Family' brother Geo. IV and William IV – a man of superior talent and decidedly liberal in his principles. His literary and scientific acquirements are great. He is one of the tallest and stoutest men in the kingdom, he is corpulent and pot-bellied, something peculiarly jolly in his appearance. Age 45.

Memoirs of Lope de Vega and several other works, as well as translating several Spanish plays. His home in Kensington was for a long time, a hospitable resort for distinguished men of literature and politics.

[125] Third Marquis of Lansdowne. He first studied in Edinburgh and later at Cambridge, finalising his education with a Continental tour. He soon entered the House of Commons and later, as Lord Henry Petty, he became a prominent Whig and Chancellor of the Exchequer. In both houses of Parliament he was a strong advocate for the abolition of slavery and also for the repeal of the penal laws against Roman Catholics. He was not a member of Wellington's party and was the Opposition leader of the House of Lords during Sir Robert Peel's rule.

[126] Lord Duncannon, John William Ponsonby. Graduated Christ Church Oxford 1802 MA.

[127] Duke of Sussex (1773-1861) also Duke of Brunswick-Luneburg. It is said that he was one of the few who cheered at the coronation of Queen Victoria.

Duke of Sutherland[128] – Great weight among the Liberal party with the exception of Marquis of Westminster, the richest peer in the realm annual income 300,000 pounds. Age 50.

Liberal Party Marquises –
The Marquis of Westminster[129], late Earl of Grosvernor – well known for the liberality of his political opinion. The richest individuals in the empire, little short of that of Sovereign – about 1000 pounds per day. And from the growing value of his houses in Pimlico, in a few years will be 500,000 pounds per annum about the Royalty itself.

Marquis of Arylesea[130], late Lord Lieutenant of Ireland, possesses considerable talent. Lost a leg.

Marquis of Clauricarde[131], a son in law of the late Mr Canning, is one of the most promising of the younger member of the peerage.

The Marquis of Conyngham[132] – known more from the prominent place his mother occupied in Court of George IV

---

[128] George Granville (1786-1861) graduated from Oxford. A trustee of the National Gallery of Art (1835) and until his death, also a trustee of the British Museum.

[129] Robert Grosvernor (1767-1845), 2nd Earl Grosvernor and 1st Marquis of Westminster created by William IV in 1831. A man of taste, he had a large picture gallery; was active in public affairs; the owner of famous race horses; and owner developer of considerable land in London (Belgravia).

[130] Marquis of Anglesey (1768-1854) Commander of Cavalry and Horse Artillery under the Duke of Wellington. He received a wound in his knee from one of the last shots fired. His leg was amputated and was buried at Waterloo; the grave is marked by a monument.

[131] Charles John Canning (1812-1862), Marquis of Clauricarde. He entered Parliament in 1836; and later served as Governor of India.

[132] Marquis of Conyngham (1766-1832?) if the date of death is correct, he would not have been in the House of Lords when JSC visited. His mother had served King George IV who lavished presents on her and the family. Their influence ended with his death.

than from anything that he has said or done himself, quite a dandy in his time.

Liberal Party, Earls -

Earl Grey[133] – celebrated for his support of liberal principles – as the author of Reform Bill. Great dignity, much of the aristocrat. He is somewhat above the middle size, eye's small forehead finely developed.

Lord Durham[134], is the great and only hope of this movement party – formerly John Geo. Lambton. Decided radical – framer of the first reform bill – son in law of Lord Grey, age 44.

The Earl of Radnor is another radical – more so than Lord Durham – friend and admirer of Cobbett. Talent about mediocrity.

---

[133] Charles Earl Grey (1764-1845) was educated at Eton, Cambridge and by a Continental tour. On his return in 1786 he became a member of Parliament, took the liberal side, and in 1792 helped found the 'Society of the Friends of the People'. He strongly supported the act to abolish the slave trade. At the death of his father he became Lord Grey and moved to the House of Lords as one of the Opposition leaders. King William IV called upon him to form a new cabinet after the fall of Wellington, so he became Prime Minister. His policy was, 'Peace, Retrenchment and Reform'. He was in and out of power for a number of years, depending on the party in control.

[134] Lord Durham was Eton educated and at the age of twenty-one became a Member of Parliament for the county of Durham. In 1828 he became a Baron and two years later was made Lord Privy Seal under Earl Grey. In 1833 he was sent to Russia on a special mission and in 1835 was sent for a second time; he became a favourite of the Emperor. In 1838 he was sent to Canada as Governor-General, but soon returned because he did not feel he had the support of his own government. This was the close of his public life.

Earl of Carnarvon[135] – is a young man of great promise – fine speaker – age 36.

Earl of Mulgrave[136] – the present Lord Lieutenant of Ireland, is a nobleman of considerable talents and highly cultivated mind.

Barons –

Lord Brougham[137] – lofty forehead dark complexion – prominent nose – dark grey hair – attenuated appearance altogether. His mind is gigantic – his industry untiring & knowledge almost boundless – his temper is very hot and hasty

---

[135] Henry John George Herbert (1800-1849) was the 3rd Earl of Carnarvon. Educated at Eton he attended Christ Church college, Oxford, but he did not graduate. He loved adventure so travelled to Portugal, Spain and Greece. He wrote and published poems and books on Spain. He opposed Liberal measures in House of Lords. In his private life he was very kind and unassuming.

[136] Earl of Mulgrave, Constantine Henry Phipps (1797-1863) was a member of the House of Commons after College 1818. He succeeded his father as an Earl and was appointed Governor of Jamaica. He held many important positions throughout his political life, including Ambassador to Paris.

[137] Lord Henry Brougham was educated in the High School and University of Edinburgh and quickly distinguished himself in the field of Mathematics. Although determined to become a lawyer, he spent considerable time travelling on the continent, and upon his return he was admitted to the Society of Advocates. He became a contributor to the *Edinburgh Review* and had several books published. In 1807 he moved to London and quickly qualified for the Bar, and by 1810 he had become a member of the Parliament, a Whig. After a four year absence from Parliament, he came back in 1816 and by 1820 was called upon to defend Queen Caroline against her husband George IV. By 1830, under Earl Grey, he became Lord Chancellor; however, after four years a change of leadership excluded him from the government. With a pension of five thousand pounds per year, as well as his other resources as an attorney and writer, he was able to live a very full life until the age of ninety.

– wants discretion – the creature of impulse – but his most splendid oratorical efforts have been made under the dominion of the most angry feelings. His presence of mind in such cases never deserts him. His moral code is great! Nothing can daunt him. He is proud and overbearing, his whole demeanour shows how conscious he is of his own surprising (?) powers. As a writer in periodicals one of the most voluminous of the day. Edinburgh Review amount to the amount of 10 or 12 volumes. British and Foreign Review. Age 57.

Lord Plunkett[138] – a man of high abilities. Dextrous debate, but as a mere speaker he does not rank high-bred to the law his features indicate cunning, ill natured & selfishness.

Lord Cottenham[139] present Lord Chancellor.

Lord Langdale formerly Mr Bicker Steth – was master of the Rolls – originally destined to the Med.Pros. married the Countess of Oxford's daughter, and applied himself successfully to the law (at 50).

Lord Hatherton[140] – Well known formerly as Mr Littleton – Secretary for Ireland under the ministry of Earl Grey, Age 45.

---

[138] William Conyngham Plunkett, first Lord, Irish lawyer and statesman, distinguished himself by his oratorical talents while a student at Trinity College. By 1787 he was admitted to the Bar and within twenty years had accumulated a large fortune and appointment to the House of Commons, a Whig. Seven years later he was Lord Chief Justice of Commons Pleas of Ireland and a peer of the United Kingdom. During the passage of the Roman Catholic Emancipation Bill, he was a constant advisor to the Duke of Wellington in the House of Lords. Later he became Chancellor of Ireland for eleven years before retiring to his estate in Ireland. Although compared with Pitt and Burke as orators, it is said that this was true as an attorney, but not in the area of Legislation: his background was not adequate.

[139] Charles Christopher Pepys was created Baron Cottenham 16 January, 1836 and took his seat in the House of Lords in February. As a lawyer he soon brought in bills for the better administration of Justice. Lord Campbell said that his speeches were confused and dissuasive, and both bills failed.

Neutral Peers -
Duke of Richmond - and Earl of Ripon, formerly Mr Robinson.

Lords, Spiritual -
Dr Wm. Howley[141], Archbishop of Canterbury, Primate of all England - not a man of any grasp or vigour of mind.

Dr Whateley[142], Archbishop of Dublin is better known as an author, than as a legislator. Thinks the moral law was superseded by the Christian dispensation & consequently not binding on Christians. In politics he is liberal.

Dr Philpots[143], Bishop of Exeter, most talented man on the Bench of Rt.Rev... (?) eloquent.

---

[140] Edward John Littleton, Lord Hetherton was a supporter of the Roman Catholic church. He was a man of moderate abilities but of unimpeachable character. He was created a Baron in 1835 and took a seat in the House of Lords immediately.

[141] William Howley (1766-1848) was educated at Winchester School and Oxford (with honours). In 1809 he was appointed Professor of Divinity. He tutored the Prince of Orange and later William II of Holland, 1813. He was nominated Bishop of London for fifteen years, seldom took part in secular discussions in the House of Lords and opposed the Catholic Emancipation Bill in 1829.

[142] Dr Richard Whatley had a distinguished career at Oxford. In 1831 he was consecrated as Archbishop of Dublin. He wrote voluminously, including, *The Elements of Logic, The Elements of Rhetoric, Introductory Lectures Upon St Pauls Epistles, Lectures on Political Economy* and *Historical Doubts Relative to Napoleon Bonaparte*.

[143] The Rt Rev Henry Philpots, DD for thirty-nine years Bishop of Exeter. He was educated at Cathedral School, Gloucester, and Corpus Christi, College, Oxford. He was ordained in 1803. In 1828 he was made Dean of Chester by Duke of Wellington (1830 became Bishop of Exeter). An able debater and an earnest churchman, he was somewhat intolerant of oppositions views and equally opposed to Romanism and Calvinism.

Dr Bloomfield[144], Bishop of London – leader of the Evangelical party – has one rule for the rich and other for the poor.

Dr Maltby[145], Bishop of Durham – decidedly liberal.

Bishop of Hereford – Brother of Earl Grey.

Saturday, September 24th, 1836 – Wrote yesterday to Camilla & took the letter to the N.C.H. but was one day too late – it will not go before the first of Oct. Papers from New York up to the 25th Aug. Called at Mr G. Eccles & took him the proof copy corrected of the 2nd Edition of my *Remarks*. Also, put on two bandages and pads on his children.

Sunday, September 25th – went to see Mr Woodward, City Road and from thence walked around by Islington[146] through Tavistock Sq. to Sacksville St.

Monday, September 26th – On Saturday last I went to Covent Garden Theatre with a friend, to see Chas Kemble[147] in

---

[144] Chas James Bloomfield (1786-1857) Bishop of London, was a writer as well as religious leader. He was an effective speaker especially on ecclesiastical subjects. His son and biographer became suffragan Bishop of Colchester in 1882.

[145] Edward Malthy (1770-1859), was the son of a master weaver and deacon in the Presbyterian Church. The son became Bishop of Chichester and later of Durham. He was active in securing a charter ·for Durham University in 1837, to which he left his library. He was Senator of London University.

[146] Islington, when JSC visited, was largely dairy farms, but is now a crowded part of London.

[147] Charles Kemble, was the father of Fanny Kemble who in 1838 came to America and married the son of a prominent Philadelphian. Her father and mother were the most celebrated family of actors in England. Charles' father had been a strolling player, and eight of his children achieved varying degrees of success as actors and theatrical managers. Charles Kemble achieved his fame as a Shakespearean

that character of Shylock – it was the first time I had seen him perform. He has some good points, but I do not consider him by any means a first rate performer. An act of *Zazezizozn*[148] was performed – laughable affair – City of Dominoes – Concluded with the play of Robt. Maccaire.

Wednesday, Sept. 28th – Read last evening a work in 2 Vol. entitled, Edrich V. Saxon. Miserable trash. Recd. a letter from Camilla dated Aug. 28th.

Friday, 30th – Revd. of Mr. Eccles 50 copies *Remarks*. Revd. of H. Bickes 18s for two doz. pamphlets sold by him and sent him two dozen of 2nd Edition.
A person called and bought a pamphlet.

Saturday, October 1, 1836 – Went to the Olympic Theatre[149] – of which Mme Vestris is the manager. It is small but got up in very good taste – the boxes are decorated with crimson curtains & are very comfortable. The performances were

---

actor. This might have been his farewell appearance on the London stage. The theatre JSC attended was on the site of the first Covent Garden built by Richard, the Harlequin, in 1732 and rebuilt after a disastrous fire (1808-1809) in which twenty three firemen lost their lives. In this second theatre, Handel produced THE MESSIAH six years after JSC's visit London. This theatre was also burned to the ground in 1856 and was rebuilt two years later as the Royal Opera House. In 1946 it became the National Royal Opera House.

[148] *Zazezizozn* may be derived from *Zarzelon*, a Spanish operetta.

[149] The Olympic Theatre opened September 1806 as the Olympic Pavilion and in 1813 as the Olympic Theatre. When Eliza Vestris took over as manager, the theatre became very fashionable. Mme Vestris was a clever actress and singer, the first woman theatre manager. She featured John Liston and Charles James Matthews whom she eventually married, although he was seven years younger. The theatre burned to the ground in 1849 but was rebuilt; it closed permanently in 1897.

Court favours the old and young Stager – Forty and Fifty – Liston[150] appeared in the two last. He is an excellent comic actor; his excellence does not consist so much in what he says as in the manner, the look, the expression – he is perfectly natural – no effort no straining for wit – no forced labour endeavour to make the audience laugh. Madam Vestris is also an excellent actress; a fine looking woman with apparently a great deal of good sense.

One peculiarity of this theatre is that there is no gallery – the Gods seems to be banished from Olympus.

Monday, 2nd, 1836 – Went to Covent Garden to witness MacCready's performance in the character of Macbeth. It was the first time I had seen that tragedy acted and the first time of my seeing MacCread – I was pleased with his performance. His combat with McDuff was particularly fine.

Thursday, 6th, 1836 – On Tuesday last I went to The Hunterian School of Medicine – so called from the building having been occupied formerly by the great John Hunter[151] –

---

[150] John Liston was a very popular actor of low comedy, whose natural humour and talent afforded many treats for London theatre goers. Early in his career, Charles Kemble recognised his ability as an actor and recommended him to the manager of the Haymarket Theatre where he frequently appeared. He played a number of theatres in London 1805-1831 but tempted by an offer of a hundred pounds per week by Mme Vestris at the Olympic Theatre, he remained for six years, which closed his acting career. He died in 1846 a wealthy man.

[151] John Hunter and his brother William were well known physicians in the 18th century. John became a recognised authority and teacher of anatomy. He was associated with many teaching hospitals 1754-1793, including St George's. After serving in the military, in 1763 he rented a house in Golden Square, not far from Piccadilly and Regent streets, where he made more than four thousand preparations of specimens to aid in the teaching of human and comparative anatomy. These include many skeletons of animals and humans, foetus, skulls,

and heard two lectures by Mr Lucas[152] & Dr Ryan[153] – Introductory. The lectures were delivered in the room formerly occupied by the Museum of John Hunter.

Yesterday I wrote to my dear wife. How much I love her! and is she not worthy of all affection? Visited the Charing Cross Hospital[154] – heard Mr. Howshit lecture on morbid anatomy to whom I was introduced and also Dr Chowne[155] lecture on midwifing. The audience consisted of two students the house apothecary.

Went St James Theatre[156], King St, St James Square said to be the handsomest theatre in Europe. There is a great deal of carving & gilding crimson silk curtains – beautiful chandeliers and most uncomfortable seats in the pit. The acting was execrable with one exception, that of Monsieur Jacquor [?].

---

and dental samples. The facility, exhibits and classes became known as The Hunterian School. At his death in 1793, the specimens were preserved and bought by the government under King George III; when the Royal College of Surgeons added a new building to the facilities at Lincoln Inn, they were put on display again.

Unfortunately, about half of the collection was lost in a bomb explosion May 11, 1941, but the very interesting and important remains are still available for study.

[152]Dr Phillip Bennett Lucas (1804-1856), was a surgeon at Metropolitan Free Hospital and a lecturer on Principles and Practices of Surgery.

[153] Dr Ryan was a surgeon, a member of The Hunterian Society and probably with Dr Lucas. He published a book of Midwifery.

[154] Charing Cross Hospital was new when JSC was in London, it had opened with sixty beds in 1834.

[155] Dr Wm Dingle Chowne (1791-1870), one of the original managers of the medical school. He lectured on obstetrics and medicine. He was president of Westminster Medical Society and later president of the Medical Society of London.

[156] The St James' Theatre was built for a celebrated opened December 14, 1835 while JSC was in Paris. The theatre was renamed The Princess in 1840. It was closed and demolished in 1957. It has now been replaced by a block of office buildings.

Saturday 8th – Went to the Adelphi Theatre[157] in the Strand. The performances were *Novelty* – a collections of absurdities too silly to mention – 'The Doom of Marana' from *La Chete d'un Ange* of Alexander Dumas, in which the absurd – the improbable – the supernatural – the horrible and the ridiculous are mingled, without exciting interest. The conclusion 'The Wreck Ashore' was better. In it John Reeve acted the parish constable, and supported the honour of his late father the... [?] with great dignity. Buckstone[158], also performed his part well, considerable merit as a comic.

Monday, October 10th, 1836 – Some time since I went to a place Piayeya [?] Covent Garden, where nightly assemble persons connected with the theatre. Players and play goers after the performances are over (about midnight) they drop in

---

[157] The Adelphi Theatre opened in 1806. It had originally been built by a John Scott, principally as an outlet for his talented daughter. Scott sold the theatre and when it was remodelled it had gas lighting, including a gas chandelier suspended from the dome over the audience; this was universally admired. It became one of the most popular theatres. It again changed hands in 1825 and in 1831 was taken over by the English Opera Company, whose theatre had been burned. In 1833 Mme Celeste made her first appearance in a speaking part. In 1834 the first mechanical device to effect a 'Sinking Stage' was added. A contemporary writer in 1835 described the theatre "by far the most fashionable attended theatre in London." It has undergone reconstruction several times, so today nothing of the original exists except the Royal Entrance, beside the stage door on Maiden Lane. The theatre is on The Strand.

[158] John Buckstone became an actor at age 19, playing in theatres in the provinces and after a few years, he appeared at the Surrey Theatre in London. He began writing plays and appeared at the Adelphi theatre in 1828 in *Luke the Labourer*. Sir Walter Scott encouraged his writing. He wrote several pieces for the Haymarket Theatre, which hired him as a comedian for several years. He also served as manager of theatres which he leased.

here to drink and to sup. A president is appointed who sings and calls upon others to do so. In this way they drink & sing until near morning, very often. All those who frequent this place have the air of gentlemen. A long room (50 ft in length I should think) with three rows of tables even completely filled when I was there. The refreshments are the best quality & the charges high this keeps out rabbles. The singing was very fine – glee songs etc. Some of the best singers in London, it is said, frequent this place. Evans, who keeps the place – rather the place keeps him – was formerly an actor and singer of much merit.

Tuesday 11th Recd. two letters from Camilla dated Pottsville September 5th and 12th. Packet of 16th in with papers to the 19th acknowledges letters of July 15th & 27th & is aware that Mr John Sanderson[159] was about to return. Papers mention the death Aaron Burr[160]. How many deaths have occurred since my departure, of celebrated men & the persons with whom I was acquainted? James Monroe[161] – Bishop White – Edw. Livingston etc, etc.

Last evening I went to the school of Medicine of St George's Hospital[162], and heard Mr Liston[163] and Dr Wilson lecture on

---

[159] Mr Sanderson was JSC's father-in-law, who was en route home.

[160] Aaron Burr, Vice President to President Jefferson, had killed Alexander Hamilton in a duel in 1804. This ended Burr's political career.

[161] President James Monroe (1751-1831), was the 5th President of the United States. (This death occurred four years before JSC travelled to France and England).

[162] St George's Hospital, from 1734 until the present century, was located at Hyde Park Corner, originally in a group of houses, three floors and a basement. A new hospital had been built in 1834 and a medical school had started in 1831. More recently the hospital and medical school have been moved a considerable distance across the Thames, south to Tooting Broadway, an area which is very much in need of hospital facilities.

surgery and physic. Liston is a canny Scott, who has obtained considerable celebrity as a surgeon, but he is a wretched lecturer. I was introduced to him, and he appears to be full of good nature. Wilson is an opponent of Pathology[164] and dislikes names. He thinks with Chapman that names are things and thinks we should avoid the influence of nosology[165] and look only at the disease.

Today I heard Mr Lucas on anatomy and Dr Lane on medicine at The Hunterian School of Medicine.

Wednesday, October 12, 1836 – Packet of the 24 Sept. has arrived. Very short passage. I have been much interested in reading the *Memoirs of the Duchess D'Abantes*, widow of Qunor. Her work in 8 Vols. Octavo, throws a great deal of light on the character on Napoleon and his family and of many of those who figure largely under the government of Bonaparte. She appears to be a woman of spirit and talent and her society is still sought after & her soirees last winter, when I was in Paris, were considered among the most agreeable in that city. She possesses a vast fund of information and anecdote and a knowledge of persons, which, her pleasing manner of conversing, makes her society sought after.

---

[163] Robert Liston (1794-1747), after finishing college, took up residence in Edinburgh and quickly "rose to the highest eminence both as a lecturer and operator." His fame quickly spread and he was much in demand as a surgeon and a lecturer in medical schools throughout England. Unfortunately, he was not a good lecturer, but was famous for his dexterity with the knife. He wrote *Principles of Surgery* in 1833. Dr Liston died suddenly at the age of fifty-four.

[164] Pathology – the study of the essential nature of diseases and especially the structural and functional changes produced by them.

[165] Nosology – a branch of medicine which deals with classification or list of diseases.

Heard Mr Lane lecture – went to the Middlesex Hospital to hear Dr Mayo[166], but he sent an excuse to his class. From thence I went to the London University Med. School and heard Mr Sam Cooper[167], author of the *Surgical Dictionary* lecture.

Met Dr Black in Fleet St. 162 – conduct a newspaper of 'uncompromising liberal principles' called the *Constitutional* promised to send me a patient.

Last night heard Mr Wardsop[168] lecture on surgery and Dr Lane on Medical Jurisprudence, at The Hunterian school.

Dined again after a considerable interval at 333 Strand. There is a table d'hote at 5 1/2 o'clock. Two kinds of excellent soup (oxtail and mock turtle) boiled salmon & stewed eels – roast duck, roast mutton, boiled pork roast, fowls, and roast shoulder of venison with salad and bread and cheese constituted the dinner – price 1s 6d.

Tuesday, 18 October, 1836 – On Friday last, the fourteenth day of October I entered on my thirtieth year. On the twentieth inst. I will be exactly one year since I left Phila.

How well I do remember the day & the circumstances, the passage in the steamboat from Phila. to New Castle, the breakfast on board – my wife & children and Susan. The Hotel at New Castle where Mr Price and Mrs S. and Mr Price had come to meet us & take leave of me. Poor Matilda! She got

---

[166] This was not the Dr Mayo of the famous present day American medical clinics.

[167] Dr Sam Cooper (1781-1848) served as a surgeon during the Battle of Waterloo. He became a professor of surgery at University College in 1831. He was a Hunterian lecturer. Writing the Dictionary was a monumental task and he had no assistance in writing the book. It became a text for every student of surgery.

[168] James Wardrop (1782-1869) a Scotsman who came to London in 1801, but four years later returned to Edinburgh until 1808. He was Surgeon Extra Ordinary to the Prince Regent (1823), and when the Prince became King George IV in 1828 he was given a title. He did not have a good reputation as a lecturer.

out of a sick bed to come and see me and has not been well since. I love her as much as if she were my own sister. And then the parting, the hurried farewell, the hasty kiss – the long embrace of my dear wife and children – and my boy, my beautiful, my bright how he cried to go with his Papa! I have never forgotten his piteous cries for his Papa. I would that I were once more at home that I might, while listening to the wind moaning around the corners of the house & signing among the solemn Pines, draw to my heart, her whom my soul loveth with the children of our affection. Oh to know the true value of a wife and children and home and friends, it is necessary to be separated from them – to be thrown among strangers in a strange land.

Last night Edwin Forrest[169] made his first appearance on a European stage at Drury Lane, in the character of Spartacus. The gladiator, I believe is the first American tragedy ever performed on this side of the Atlantic. Forrest was received with great applause and his debut may be considered as highly successful & flattering. The House was full. After the fall of the curtain he was loudly called for – he made his appearance & addressed the audience in a brief speech thanking them for the kind reception his 'humble efforts' and for the reception of the tragedy of Dr Bird his friend. To the latter part there was some dissent.

Wednesday, 19th October, 1836 – The daily press, so far as I have seen it, speaks in high terms of Forrest and his performance but pretty generally censure the Play. *The Times*

---

[169] Edwin Forrest was a prominent American actor who encouraged American playwrights. A review in *John Bull* newspaper the next day was excellent; "more enthusiasm we have hardly seen"; the October 30 edition of the same paper said "by particular desire a repeat performance by E Forrest." The COURIER gave the actor a great review the next day; "a success as triumphant as could have been desired by his most enthusiastic admirers".

says that, 'his performance during the whole of the last act was a blaze of splendour'. The thing is settled – his debut has been highly satisfactory.

I'm reading the *Metropolitan Magazine*[170] for October. I met with article headed Letter to Brother John, No.8 By E. Johnson, with, which I was very much pleased. Not as containing anything new, but as embodying ideas & doctrines which I have long since acted upon in practice – and which are expressed in a clear and forcible manner.

Friday, 21st October – Yesterday a year ago, I left Phila. & embarked at New Castle on board the Algonquin for Liverpool. When shall I return? That is concealed in the dark womb of time – Clouds and darkness rest upon it. It is now nearly two weeks since I have had a letter from Camilla, and I am anxious to hear from her and to learn that her father[171] has safely reached his home.

Sunday, October 23rd, 1836 – There have been a few days this month tolerable pleasant and this day in Particular – warm, smoky, sunshiny day. The air was delightful. Dr Carrol and myself walked out through the Regents Park[172], by the

---

[170] *Metropolitan Magazine* for September 15, 1836 contained the article 'Letters to Brother John' by E Johnson. The letters describes a condition of the body in which, "no actual disease can be said to exist". He concludes by describing the difficulty as "indigestion, a condition from which few people are free". In the October issue of the magazine the letter continues and concludes that "a sleepy, feeble, and inefficient circulation is brought on by the lazy life we lead." The October issue also contained an article on Phrenology.

[171] Mr Sanderson had been to London before leaving for home.

[172] Regent's Park is a nearly circular area of four hundred and seventy acres, well designed and landscaped with lakes, open fields, shrubbery and flowers. The park is surrounded by buildings. At the northern extremity of the park is the Zoological Gardens, opened in 1826. The zoo is quite extensive and beautifully planned and landscaped.

Zoological Gardens to Primrose Hill. From the top of this hill we would have had a fine view of London if the atmosphere had been clear, a circumstance that very rarely occurs in London. As it was, the view was delightful. On one side the mighty city of London lay hushed in the calm of the Sabbath – more immediately under the eve, in the same direction, Regents

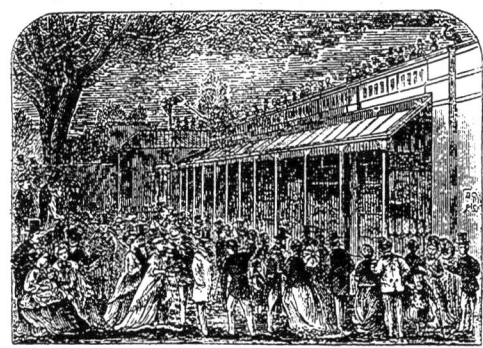

Zoological Gardens

Park with the Zoological Gardens, crowded with well dressed people – on the opposite side of the hill Thackery, Kentish house and various other villages with their churches and steeples pointing to the sky from amongst the trees, and whose bells tolled the good people to prayers – the numerous & beautiful country residences in every direction – the rich green sward – all spoke beauty and delight to senses.

Last night went to the St Bartholomew's Hospital[173] Smithfields, and heard Dr Latham[174] lecture on the pulse, the

---

[173] The St Bartholomew's Hospital was founded in 1123 by Rahere, an Augustinian canon. It was run by monks and sisters. The present hospital building is Georgian and was designed by James Gibbs in 1702. Hogarth, the English artist, was a life governor of the hospital since he provided paintings for the hospital, including the large painting on the walls of the main stairway. Today the hospital has six hundred and eighty beds, but presently its future is threatened by cuts in government spending.

hard & soft – the small & full or large pulse. He laid great stress on the hard pulse, as an indication of organic disease or inflammation and as a guide for V.S. Seldom dares to bleed when that is absent & seldom withholds it when present. This hospital is said to be the largest in London.

Monday, 24 October, 1836 – One of my patients residing at Norwich, sent me a basket of game as a present, a hare a brace of pheasant and a brace of partridges some nuts – I sent the hares and a pheasant to Mr Todhunter.

Went to King's College[175] and heard Mr Arnott[176], lecture on surgery. Erysipelos, phlegm furonclus, Carbuncle & ulceration.

Wednesday, October 26th – This evening went to the Hunterian school heard Mr. Wardrop – showed us a cancerous

---

[174] Peter Mere Latham (1789-1875), graduated from Oxford with an MD in 1816. After continued study, he was admitted to the College of Physicians in 1818 (he was attached to Middlesex Hospital at the time). In 1824 he was appointed physician to St Bartholomew's Hospital where he contributed to improving the medical school. His lectures were enthusiastically received. Sir Thomas Watson said in 1836 when some of his lectures were published, "The publications marked an area in the clinical teaching of this country." Dr Latham later published two volumes of *Lectures on Diseases of the Heart*. His health had always been delicate (emphysema of the lungs and asthma) and consequently he left the work at the hospital in 1845. He continued his practice of medicine until he retired in 1865.

[175] King's College is located in The Strand adjacent to Somerset House (government offices) near Waterloo Bridge.

[176] Dr Neil Arnott (1794-1885) a Scotsman, invented the water-bed and floating mattress for patients with acute suffering. He also invented the Arnott's Stone and Arnott's Ventilator. He received many honours over the years, including the Cross of the Legion of Honour awarded by Napoleon III. He was a member of the Council, Royal College of Surgeons and Surgeon Extra Ordinary to the Dowager Queen, and Professor of Surgery at King's College in 1836.

tumour afterwards went to the Blenheim school and heard Mr Marshal Hall[177] on the nervous system. Read an excellent review of Dr Latham's work. *Auscultation* must get the work.

Thursday 27th – Yesterday and today I went to the Westminster School of Med.[178] to hear Mr Gutherie[179] – but for some cause, he did not lecture and this evening I went to King's College and heard Dr Wilson[180] on the termination of inflammations. The professors of this college wear gowns.

Friday, October 28th – Yesterday I wrote to Dr Tucker, and Recd. a letter from Camilla, my dear boy was not well and little Sally had scalded herself – how careful we should be to place things beyond the reach of children – especially such as are liable to burn or scald – from a little accident like that which

---

[177] Marshall Hall (1790-1857), a graduate of the University of Edinburgh was later house physician at the Edinburgh Royal Infirmary 1812. He studied in Paris, Göttingen, and Berlin. In 1825 he was appointed physician to Nottingham General Hospital where he achieved fame for his research. He published papers included *Diseases of Females*. Hall is credited with discovering 'reflex action' but not without controversy. He was more highly regarded abroad than in London in the beginning. Another of his publications was *Principles of Pathology in the Nervous System*.

[178] Westminster School of Medicine was established in 1719.

[179] Dr George James Gutherie (1785-1856) passed examinations for The Royal College of Surgeons in 1801 before he was sixteen. He founded an infirmary for eye diseases which afterwards became The Royal Westminster Ophthalmic Hospital. Elected a full surgeon in 1827, he was a very popular lecturer interspersing his subject with anecdotes and illustrative cases. JSC may have heard his lecture, 'The Anatomy and Diseases of the Urinary and Sex Organs', which he delivered in 1836. Many of his lectures and papers have been published. His son succeeded him in 1843.

[180] The Doctor Wilson, JSC heard may have been Sir William Erasmus Wilson (1809-1884). He wrote many papers on dermatology.

only lightly scalded my child, she might, had the cocoa been hotter, have been horribly deformed all her life. Letter dated 27 Sept. and came by the Packet of the first. Mr Sanderson has not arrived – but she mentioned the packet of the 21st Aug. as in from Liverpool – that I have known ten day or two weeks – strange that the Havre packets should be so far behind.

Saturday 29th – Wrote to Camilla and walked to the North and South American Coffee house to put the letter in the mail bag for Portsmouth.

Read James new work *The Desultory Air*. It consists of a variety of detached thesis loosely connected by the appearance of a general tale. The work has the look of being made up with but slender material.

Monday, 31st October, 1836 – Yesterday went to St Martins in the Field Church[181] heard a good sermon. Took tea with Dr Carrol and had a long discussion with him on the subject of religion. He is a decided infidel.

Revd. two letters from Dr Tucker, Paris, this morning dated October 27th and 29th in which he makes some propositions with the regard to the payments of his notes which did not enter into the scope of our agreement. Answered these propositions and accepted them conditionally. To give me five hundred Franks cash and the same sum every three months provided 1/2 the profits do not exceed that sum – if they do I am to have the benefit of that excess [?] that is one half the profits.

Went to hear Mr McDermott lecture, Gerard St. School of Med[182] not being well he merely ground them.

---

[181] St Martin-in-the-Fields was begun in 1721 and finished five years later, but it had been preceded by an earlier church during the reign of Henry VIII. Gibbs was the architect. Nell Gwynne is buried in the churchyard, and a number of royal babies have been christened in this church.

Afterwards went to Westminster School of Med. and heard Mr Gutherie lecture, or rather talk on surgery.

'That the mind of desultory man,
Studious of change & pleased with novelty,
May be indulged.'

The author of *The Diary of a Physician* is Mr Warren[183] an English barrister, son of Dr Warren.

An apothecary charged a family of seven persons 149 pounds for medicine furnished during one year and a half – forty-two shillings worth of medicine was charged in one day[184].

Tuesday, November 1, 1836 – Read Capt. Chamier[185] novel *Ben Brace – The Last of the Agamemnons*. It is a true sailor's yarn. Ben from his youth upward was attached to Nelson & became a mongrel kind of clerk to him: part servant, part valet, part Secretary, and all sailor. Under this character, Capt.

---

[182] Gerard Street School of Medicine may have been mainly for treatment of the eyes.

[183] Samuel Warren (1807-1877) studied medicine in Edinburgh, then turned to law and was called to the bar from the Inner Temple in 1837. He wrote a number of technical legal works, and became a Queen's Counsel in 1851. In 1853 he was given an honorary doctorate at Oxford. He served three years in Parliament. Many of his writings were published anonymously, including *The Dairy of a Late Physician,* which was attributed to a well known doctor who was charged with betraying medical secrets. His best known novel, *Ten Thousand a Year* was extremely popular when first published.

[184] Approximately $670 a year. $9.66 per day.

[185] Frederick Chamier 1796-1870 entered the Royal Navy in 1808 and was promoted to Lieutenant by 1815, serving in the Mediterranean and the West Indies. 1826 he was appointed Commander. He retired in 1833, but was given the rank of Captain in 1856. He devoted his retired life to writing mostly sea stories. *Ben Brace* was published in 1836.

Chamier has continued to give a great many particulars of Britain's naval hero, not generally known.

Saturday, November 5, 1836 – Yesterday Mr Eccles called and invited me to take supper with him this evening at 8 o'clock.

Heard Mr. Wardrop lecture this evening on the treatment of wounds.

Sunday November 6, 1836.   Last night being the anniversary of the Gun Powder Plot – there was a great waste of powder in the form of squibs rockets *et hoc genusomnes*. Something of the same kind as that which occurs on New Year's Eve.

Went to Mr Eccles where we had *une petite soupe*. The company was composed of two lectures in a gratuitous School of Med.

After supper we had a drink made of ale, eggs, & spirits, which they call Flip – it is drunk hot.

Went to St George's chapel[186] Regency St. It is very pretty & very capacious building surmounted with a dome & lantern which is supported by four arches. It has two galleries on each side of it – the pews of all the churches that I have been in are high and strait backed, as in our old churches. The pulpit is placed near the middle of the building to one side, sometimes a reading desk is on one side & the pupil on the other.

Monday, 7th November, 1836 – This morning I recd. two letters from the U.S.– one from Camilla dated October 12,

---

[186] St George Church was built between 1720-1724 and designed by a pupil of Gibbs, John James.   Some of the windows contain early Renaissance stained glass (installed after JSC's visit).   Today the church is the scene of fashionable weddings in addition to the regular services.

Pottsville, the other from Cornelia[187] dated Brandywine Oct. 9. She mentions the arrival of Mr Sanderson, who landed about the lst of the same month, well and safely though he narrowly escaped drowning in going from the ship to the land in a steamboat, in consequence of a storm. Cornelia has not received my letter, strange. She writes a very good letter & knows my weak side, she flatters me in praising my children, Johnny is a genius and Sally a beauty. But parents like to be flattered on that subject even when they know it to be flattery – though I have to tell the truth, some such opinion as that myself.

I have been looking through the first volume of the memories of Tucien or Lucien [?] Bonaparte, prince of Canino[188], but did not find them very interesting. They consist principally of legislative discussions, speeches and etc. nearly glancing at the military operations as they were connected with the civil power.

Dined with Mr W. Eccles at Short's Grand Hotel and promised to take breakfast with him on Wednesday morning at 10 o'clock, after which we are to go and gaze at the Lord Mayor's pageant, it being Lord Mayor's Day.

Heard Mr Wardrop lecture – treatment of punctured wounds.

Tuesday, November 8, 1836 – Went to hear Dr Ryan at The Hunterian School lecture. Dr Ryan is editor of the London Medical and Surgical Journal – has published a manual & a treatise on obstetrics etc. He is an Irishman – has been in difficulty with his publisher and been imprisoned from whence

---

[187] Cornelia Sanderson was the sister of JSC's wife, Camilla.

[188] Lucien Bonaparte (1775-1857) was the third son of Napoleon Bonaparte. He was made Prince of Canino in 1808. On his way to America in 1810, he was taken prisoner by the English and retained for three years. After 1814 he retired to Italy. He possessed great boldness and talent.

he has just been set free. Also heard Dr Grant[189] on Comparative Anatomy – celebrated man Scotsman. Mr Ward also lectured this evening on Morbid Anatomy. The Arabs, says Mr. Wardrop, tie the spermatic cord leaving out the _vas deferens_ [?], by which they take away the passion without injury to the vigour of the horse and he recommends the same plan in certain cases of injury to the spermatic cord in men.

Wednesday, November 9, 1836 – Took breakfast with Mr W. Eccles and went with him afterwards to witness the procession of the Lord Mayor going to Westminster Hall[190] to take the oath of office. There were a great profusion of Flags, musicians, etc. The Sheriffs, the old and the new Lord Mayors in carriages drawn by six horses, covered with gold & silk. Men in ancient armour, city guards, etc., made up the procession – at Blackfriars Bridge they entered the city barges and were rowed to Westminster. Cannons were fired during their embarkation and progressed along the river. An immense crowd of people filled the streets, the windows and even the top of the houses. I must not forget to mention an admirable figure

---

[189] Dr Robert Edward Grant was a member of the faculty of Westminster College of London. He had many publications on anatomy as well as lectures on both human and animal anatomy.

[190] Westminster Hall is part of the old Royal Palace of Westminster. It was built during the time of William II and served as the seat of Parliament at various times and also as the seat of the law courts from the early thirteenth century until the late nineteenth century. Charles I was condemned to death in this Hall. It was the scene of Coronation Banquets until the time of George IV. It was used at one time by the House of Lords as well as the House of Commons and in various ways. Parliament continued to use the hall until 1834. Just before JSC went to London a fire swept through the old palace and the Hall. Nearly three hundred feet long, seventy feet wide and almost one hundred feet tall, the Hall is one of the largest in the world supported by pillars.

of Jim Crow which closed the procession, making an admirable burlesque of the Pageantry,

Thursday 10th – heard Ryan, Wardrop and M. Hall lecture yesterday; and this day in addition heard Professor Grant on Comparative Anatomy. Mr Lucas introduced me to Dr Ryan. He says he has great esteem for the Americans that he corresponds with – thinks them very clever. Alluded to Dew [?] work on midwifery in high terms of praise in his lecture this evening, and spoke of the Americans in very flattering terms to his class, and told them that there was an American gentleman in the room with whom he had the pleasure of being acquainted.

Sunday 13th – On my way from the City Road to Tavistock Sq. Passed by St Johns gate[191] which with Temple Bar, are the only remains of the ancient defences & boundaries of the City of London. It has a very ancient and Castellated appearance and belonged to the ancient order (of Knights of Jerusalem) of St John.

Monday, November 14, 1836 – Received a letter from Mr and Mrs Sanderson[192] dated Brandywine, Oct. 15. & the P.S.

---

[191] St John's Gate was the south entrance to the priory of the Knights Hospitalers of the Order of St John of Jerusalem. The Priory was founded in 1130. The Knights of St John were the soldiers of Christendom for centuries. After Queen Elizabeth suppressed the priory, it became the residence of many famous occupants, including the Master of the Revels, who licensed thirty of Shakespeare's plays. Dr Johnson was here in 1737 in a room, and started his literary career. In 1745 the Gate became The Jerusalem public-house, and in 1845 it was restored. Today is it a depository for many relics of the Knights of St John.

[192] Mr and Mrs Sanderson were JSC's in-laws. Mr Sanderson had returned from Paris just a few months earlier.

of Mr S. Phila. October 18th was to start to Pottsville on the 19th.

Wednesday 16th – Yesterday I dined with Mr W. Eccles where I met Mr Myers and Mr Davis of Graves End surgeon in the British Navy who has been in North and South America. This Mr Davis is a most irregular and eccentric character. The organs of gaiety and imagination are singularly developed, and his character, I am told, corresponds to this development. His imagination and wit are the governing powers of his mind and altogether overbalance his judgement, so much so that many of his friends think him partially deranged. He was in the Sandwich Islands with the present Lord Byson, and was well acquainted with the Rev. Mr. Stewart, the American missionary.

Thursday, November 17, 1836 – Read a little work of Mr I. Wardrop on diseased structure. Called this morning on Dr Henry Davies[193], 18 Saville Row and presented a letter of introduction from Mr Cryder, promised to send me two cases of hernia. After the lecture of Drs Grant & Ryan, I went to the Phrenological Society, whose meetings are held in the museum of The Hunterian School. Mr Hawkins in the chair, read a paper in answer to a note of the Editor of the Phrenological journal, on a paper published in that Journal giving an account of precocious child, the adopted son of Mr Hawkins.

Friday, November 18 – Called on Sir Astley Cooper[194] with whom I had a long conversation on the subject of hernia – he promised to send his cases of rupture to be treated by me.

---

[193] Dr Henry Davis wrote on midwifery and women's diseases.

[194] Sir Ashley Cooper (1768-1841) devoted himself mostly to study and lecturing in his younger days. In 1829 he wrote *Illustrations of the Diseases of the Breast* The next year *Diseases of the Testes* and

Rode out to Herne Hill, Dulwich etc. with Mr W. Eccles: at the latter place stopped to dine at the Greyhound. There is a college at Dulwich[195] for the support of twelve old women, twelve old men, and twenty-four boys, founded and endowed by a Player by the name of Allen or Allein. The master's name must be Allen also. Behind the college which is of the Elizabethan style, is a gallery of five old paintings to which there is free admission.

We passed near the celebrated Norwood, a great haunt of the Gypsies – their headquarters indeed – also within sight of Beula Spa a watering place of a great resort in the summer by the citizens of London. Norwood is near Beula Spa.

Sunday, November 20, 1836 – Called on Mr Davis in St Martin's Lane at the old *Slaughter House*. Queer character. from thence walked to *Charter House Square* and visited the *Charter House Institution*[196]. It presents the appearance of an

---

also *The Anatomy of the Thymus Gland*. He served two terms as President of the Royal College of Surgeons.

[195] Dulwich was about five miles south of London Bridge. The distinguished actor who founded the college was Edward Allein, or Allen. Later the college was enlarged to accommodate six to seven hundred boys. The paintings mentioned were bequeathed in 1810 by Sir Francis Bourgeois and were chiefly of the Dutch and Flemish schools.

[196] Charterhouse has been a home for the poor, as JSC indicates, since 1611. However, the history of the buildings go back to 1371 when it was a Carthusian Monastery, until Henry VIII put an end to it (1538). In 1611 the wealthy Thomas Sutton founded the hospital and school to take care of poor men over sixty years of age, and also a school for about forty poor boys. It was later moved to Surrey and is a well known public school. Thackery was educated in the old building, as were Sir William Blackstone, John Wesley, John Leech and George Grote. Many of the buildings were seriously damaged in 1941 by air raid, but have been restored. Today the area is beautiful and still houses pensioners.

old, irregular map of strong buildings occupied before the time of Henry VIII as a Carthusian monastery – and arched gateway was shown us where the Abbot being rather refractory was hung by order of the King. The Property afterwards came into the possession of the Duke of Norfolk, who was executed for conspiracy & then Thomas Sutton, a very wealthy individual purchased it. He left, at his death, these buildings and other properties for the endowment of a charity for the support and education of eighty old men and forty-four boys. He died in 1611. Various additions and improvements have since been made in a more modern style but there are still many remains of the old massy [?] monastery with its low arches, gloomy portals, small & grated windows, heavy carved wainscots, curiously and quaintly wrought. In the chapel, where the arms of the Duke of Norfolk are frequently carved, is also seen the date of 1511 in this Chapel is to be seen some of the finest specimens of carved wood, and a handsome elaborate monument to the memory of Mmr. Sutton, Esq.

With a full length statue in a recumbent position, said to be a very correct likeness. A bust & marble tablet is also to be seen there to the memory of Lord Ellenborough, who was, by his own request buried in this place, where he had recd. his education. Steele, Addison and many other distinguished men, it is said, were also educated by this charity.

I must not forget to mention the politeness of the gentlemen belonging to the Institution whom we casually met and who took us over the buildings & pointed out the objects most worthy of our curiosity.

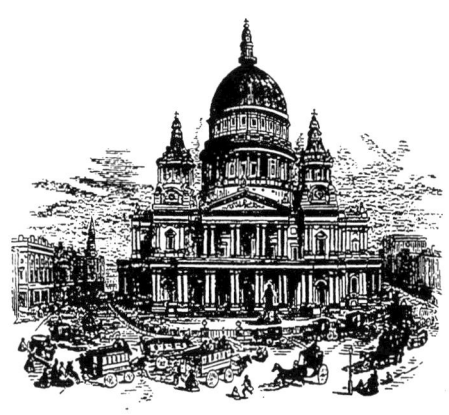

St Paul's Cathedral and Churchyard, from Ludgate Hill

Called at Mr Woodwards, City Road, and on my return stepped into Bow Church in Cheapside[197]. This church has a very fine peal of bells and it is an established opinion, that all persons born within the sound of the Bow bells are by birthright, Cockneys. Passing onward I stepped into St Paul's Cathedral[198] and listened to the music and what I could hear of

---

[197] Bow Church, St Mary-le Bow, may derive its name from the arches in the crypt beneath the church. Christopher Wren was responsible for the present church, which replaced an earlier church destroyed in the Great Fire (1666). This church is located in the area which centuries ago was the great shopping area of London. Despite the fact that most of the better shops have moved west, the area is still filled with excellent jewellers. Names of streets in the area reflect the earlier days, such as Friday Street (Friday's fish market), Milk Street, Poultry Street, Bread Street, etc. The church is close to the section of the city which today houses the great banks of England and is a short distance from St Paul's Cathedral. Standing as it does, in the centre of the city, those who are born within the sound of its bells are called Cockneys, a name equivalent to genuine citizens.

[198] St Paul's Cathedral, designed by Wren after the great fire of 1666, was the Cathedral JSC visited. It has since undergone considerable repair in the twentieth century. Wren, in designing the new church, ignored the foundations of the two older structures. Located on a hill, it is an imposing building, despite the modern buildings surrounding it

the service and the sermon, which was very little. This & the cold froze all my devotion, and I inwardly vowed as I left the building, that I would never again be caught in the fenced in portion of St Paul's during service.

Tuesday, November 22nd, 1836 – Gave notice yesterday of my intended departure.

Thursday, November 24th, 1836 – Called at the office of Mr Alban, Lincoln's Inn[199]. Mr. Chas. Dickens[200] author of Sketches of a Boy and Pickwick Club is a reporter of the *Morning Chronicle*.

Friday, November 25th, 1836 – Size of London – Length eight miles, breadth five, average breadth four do. Circumference thirty-five do population two million. Nearly doubled itself within the last half century. Yearly rental exceed seven million pounds. The only street which has any pretension to taste or beauty is Regent. Ninety thousand persons cross London Bridge in one day. London very healthy – annual

---

today. The earliest Cathedral, dating from the tenth century, was destroyed within the century. A second lasted some two hundred years. The predecessor of the present Cathedral probably was at the height of its excellence in the fifteenth century, and was destroyed by the fire of 1666. Wren's Cathedral was started in 1675 and finished in 1710, at a cost of three-quarters of a million pounds. To be noted are the magnificent domes (an outer and inner dome), the carved choir stalls, and mural decorations.

[199] Lincoln's Inn is one of the largest squares in London, dating back to the early seventeenth century. This square is surrounded today with many important buildings, such as the Royal College of Surgeons, the Old Curiosity Shop, Lincoln's Inn Library and Hall, and the Royal Courts of Justice.

[200] Charles Dickens (1812-1870) wrote under the pseudonym of 'Boz' at the time JSC was in London. His first publication, in 1836, was *Sketches By Boz* and shortly, *Pickwick Papers* in 1837.

number of deaths thirty thousand. Births exceed the annual number of deaths by two or three thousand. A hundred and twenty thousand strangers at all times in London. Scotsmen a hundred and thirty thousand – Irishmen two hundred thousand – Frenchmen thirty thousand. Twenty thousand enter daily & as many depart. Great difference in the external appearance of the people as well as in the different parts of L., metropolis of World.

Theatres, great rage for – 20,000 persons nightly attend. Number of 22. No.1 King's Theatre or Italian Opera, Haymarket four tiers of boxers & a fifth interrupted by the gallery. Mr Sams, Mr Andrews, opera book sellers speculate in opera boxes. The late Duke of Gloucester used to Pay 300 guineas every year for his box and the same sum is still payed by the Duke of Devonshire. There are no general boxes. Price to pit half guinea. Gallery 5s frequented... and... for servants of nobility. Average nightly receipts in the 800 pounds but 2,000 pounds have been taken this theatre solely confined to the presentation of Italian Opera and ballet – great place of fashionable resort – must go in full dress, cost 100,000 pounds – formerly rented for 15,000 pounds now 8,000 pounds. Only licensed for 6 months – from the last of February until August – only open 3 times a week. Thursday... night.

Drury Lane[201] Rebuilt in 1809 – cost 300,000 pounds, accommodates 3,060 persons, 5,000 been in it. Nightly expenses 180 –280 full house brings in 400 pounds but 900 has been taken – free admissions stopped in that case. Rental some

---

[201] Drury Lane, named for Sir William Drury who lived here prior to the first theatre (1663). Both this theatre and Covent Garden were burned twice prior to the nineteenth century. The present theatre opened in 1812; Byron wrote a prologue for the opening. Most of the great actors and actresses have played this theatre. The portico columns were added in 1831 and are the only part of the nineteenth century structure remaining.

years ago was 11,000 pounds lately 8,000 pounds Mr Bunn now has a lease for three years at 6,000 pounds per annum. Losses – Capt Polhill's 80,000 pounds in four years. Some years the expenditures over the income has been 30,000 pounds but in others 20,000 pounds has been gained.

Covent Garden's[202] great rival of Drury Lane rebuilt in 1809 cost 300,000 pounds – fitted up for 2,800 persons has contained 4,255. These two are called the winter houses, open nine months in the year – Oct. to July. McCready & Farren get about 30 Pounds Per week. The Material of the large theatre cost them 40,000 to 50,000 pounds each.

Haymarket – Foote, Palmer, Jack Bannister, Mathew Liston, Miss Fenton (afterwards Dutchess of Bolton) Miss Farren (present Countess of Derby) etc. made their debut at this theatre.

Clubs – two kinds. Subscription clubs, when some individual agrees to furnish all the necessary payment of a certain annual sum. The 2nd and most numerous class, is when a certain number appropriate and manage their own affairs.

Subscription – Brookes[203] St. James St, Fox, Sheraton, and etc. in numbers – White's[204], St. Jas. St. rival of Brooke's. Boodles[205], St. Jas. St... this last is a Tory, the others are Wigs.

---

[202] Covent Garden Theatre, now The Royal Opera House built in 1858, after several previous theatres.

[203] Brooke's Club was founded in 1764 as a young man's club. It has been described as 'the most famous political club that ever existed in London'. It is no longer a political club. Six to eight generations of the same family have belonged to Brooke's. Women are now permitted as guests and the 'Subscription Room' is used for debutante parties.

[204] White's Club is the oldest in London and one of the most famous in the world. It was founded in 1693 and is across the street from Brooke's. Cards are played for lower stakes than at Brooke's. Today it is one of the most financially stable of the London clubs.

The principal clubs of the 2nd class are, The Carlton, Reform, Athenaeum, Clarence, Oxford and Cambridge University Club, Oriental, Travellers Union, United Service, etc.

The Carlton Club[206] Pall Mall, decided Tory – (today 69 Pall Mall).

Reform[207] do is of recent institution (today 104 Pall Mall).

Athenaeum[208] do scientific men (today 107 Pall Mall).

Clarence do Waterloo Place is a Junior Athenaeum.

Oriental[209] Corner of Hanover Square, consists of gentlemen who have resided sometime in the east.

---

[205] Boodles, on the same street, has an air of tranquillity. Established in 1762, it was named after an early head waiter. Political involvement is not part of the club. There is a ladies' entrance in the rear.

[206] The Carlton Club, 69 St James's Street, was founded by the Duke of Wellington in 1832. Today it is the most famous political club. Many high government officials over the years have been members, including Disraeli. In 1940 the building was destroyed by a German bomb and it was moved to a former nineteenth century club building.

[207] The Reform Club, 104 Pall Mall, was founded in 1836 by a liberal and was joined by many of the Hudson Bay Company. Members of this club were considered to have radical ideas; candidates were required to express their support of the principles of the Reform Bill. Today it is not a political club, but many members are liberals. It was one of the first clubs to have bedrooms available. A very special kitchen enabled the chef to serve lavish banquets.

[208] The Athenaeum Club was founded for the intellectually and successfully elite. Some former members included Macaulay, Trollope, Matthew Arnold and Richard Burton. The club is not a place for heavy drinking and gambling, but rather a scene of genuine intellectual discussions. There is an excellent, well-maintained library.

[209] The Oriental Club on Hanover Street. It is said that Wellington advised the founders to "have a club of your own". Many 'Indians', military officers and officials of the East India Company joined.

Travellers 1(06) Pall Mall – its members must have travelled a certain distance.

Gaming Houses – Crockford's the most noted St. James Street. The largest in London – perhaps in the world – building cost 6,000 pounds, furnishings 35,000 pounds. There is nothing in London equal to the splendour of its furniture. Superb suppers are given gratis by Crockford to the members of the club. His cook is the celebrated M. Ude – salary 1,000 guinea per annum. 2nd cook gets 5,000 do per annum. The cellar from which the wines are supplied is valued at 70,000 pounds 300,000 bottles of wine besides the innumerable hogshead – 33 servants play commence at 11, doors shut at 2 – originated for the late Duke of York and some others, Crockford was originally a poor miserable fishmonger, can't read, write, or speak correctly – a large coarse vulgar looking man. Has a family of 10 children, daughter married to a clergyman.

The Times leading Journal of Europe – established 1788 edited by Mr Walter, Dr. Stoddart, and since 1815 or 16, by Mr Barnes, who has the entire conduct of the paper. Salary supposed 1,200 guineas. Mr Alsaver has for many years supplied the city article *The Times*. His salary is about 7 or 800 guineas.

In one of the double sheets of *The Times* there is a quantity of matter equal to what is contained in three ordinary octavo vols. *The Times* is estimated to be worth 250,000 pounds – 150,000 pounds of which is said to belong to the Carlton Club. Its annual profits for some years past, are supposed to be between 20,000 and 30,000 pounds. Employs directly one hundred persons – fifty or sixty compositors. Circulation 10,000.

Morning Herald Circulates 7,000 copies daily.

The *Morning Chronicle* was sold after the death of Mr Perry the former editor and proprietor to Mr Clement for 40,000 pounds. Mr Black, principal Editor, circulation about 4,500; this paper is decidedly Wig. *The Morning Post* is the organ of the fashionable world, decidedly Tory – circulation 2 or 3 thousand.

The Morning Advertiser[210], was instituted by the body Licensed Victuallers whose property it still is. By each member of this body paying 3 guineas and taking this paper daily, he becomes a proprietor and is entitled to a share of the profits. There are upward of three thousand – a certain portion of profit goes toward support & education of children of poor members of this society. Circulation five thousand daily.

The last of the morning papers is *The Public Ledger*, the oldest paper, daily, in London established in 1758. Goldsmith etc. used to write for this paper – It has lately become extinct and *The Constitutional* has risen from its ashes – thoroughly radical.

Less than 50,000 pounds would not give a chance of success in establishing a morning paper. *The Times* has paid in duty for advertisements in one year nearly twenty thousand pounds.

Evening Papers. *Globe*-ministerial, 3,000, value 50,000 pounds. *The Sun* – 3,000 copies. *The Cue Sun* (?), edited by Mr Fox – *Courier* and *The Standard* – which is the only evening Tory paper.

Weekly Papers – *Examiner* – *Spectator* – *Observer – Bell's Life in London* – this latter with the exception of *The Dispatch* has the largest circulation of any paper in the United Kingdom. *The Dispatch* has a circulation of 32,000. *Bell's Weekly Messenger*. Conservative, chiefly read in the country, circulation 13,000. *Bell's New Weekly Messenger*, *The Sunday Times*, *John Bull* – Tory Age 4,500, Tory 7250. *Satirist* 4,500 *News-Weekly*.

---

[210] The Morning Advertiser was started in 1794 and has a circulation of about 21,500.

The number of daily Journals is eleven and of the weekly 27. The aggregate circulation of the daily papers is 40,000; that of the weekly 120,000 total 160,000– 7 out of 11 dailys are liberal. There are thirteen weekly liberal papers and seven conservative. In circulation also the liberals have this ascendancy.

Quarterly Reviews -

The Quarterly Review started in 1809 by Mr Gifford and opposition to the *Edinburgh Review* – Tory in politics, circulation 9,000. Mr Gifford was succeeded by Dr Southey the poet laureate, in the editorship – and he was followed by Mr Lockhart, son in law of Sir W. Scott. Sir W. Scott reviewed his own novels in this review, in terms of high Praise. Salary of Mr Lockhart who still conducts this review is 1,400 pounds per annum. The average rate of Payment for contributions is twenty guineas for sixteen pages. This is also the price paid by *Edinburgh.*

The London and Westminster Review is radical in its politics – circulation limited – about 1,500 – is the only quarterly organ of thoroughly Liberal principles.

The Foreign Quarterly Review was started in 1823 moderately liberal circulation, below 1,200.

The British and Foreign Review, started in 1835 established by Mr Beaumont, who has an annual income 100,000 pounds. Lord Brougham has written some of its articles – decidedly liberal in politics.

The Dublin Review, appeared in April 1836 organ of the Roman Catholic – conducted by Mr. O'Connell – Dr. Wiseman and Mr McQuin decidedly liberal in political large circulation. These are the five metropolitan quarterlies.

Monthlies -
More numerous and of much greater antiquity than the Quarterlies – *Gentleman's Magazine* established in 1733 circulation of 1,200.

Monthly Review, established 1749 Smollett Goldsmith, Johnson, Sterne, Humes, Hawkesworth etc.   Contributed largely to its page.

Monthly Magazine begun in 1786 – Tory changed to Liberal.

The Eclectic Review advocates the cause of Dissent and liberal principles – partly religious and partly a literary publication.

The New Monthly Magazine – 1814 – edited by Mr Campbell & latterly by E.L. Bulever [?] and since. 1833 Mr S.C. Hall.

Frayer's Magazine. Ultra Tory.

The Metropolitan Magazine. 1831 got up in opposition to the *New Monthly Magazine*, edited by Mr. Thos. Campbell. and now by Capt. Marry at 1,500.

The Monthly Repository – organ of Unitarianism now become more political ultra liberal or rather Republican. Edited Rev. Mr Fox.

The Lady's Magazine & Museum 1755.

The Court Magazine conducted for some years by the celebrated Mrs. Norton.

The Asiatic Journal, Alexander's East India Magazine and *United Service Journals*, are the principle remaining monthlies.

Es. from *The Great Metropoles*.

Saturday, November 26th, 1836 – Finished reading *Gil Blas* in French, and I must agree with the editor of the work, that it is *pour les Francais, comme Don Quichotte pour les Espagnols, comme Tom Jones, pour les Anglais, le premier roman de la nation*. I take leave of the hero in the words of the archeveque de Granade-adieu Monsieurs Gil Blas; *je vous souhaite toutes sortes de pros perites, avec un peu (?) plus de gout.*

Bought a leather portmanteau for 13 Shillings[211].

Phrenology constitutes a part of the regular course of study, taught at the Argyll Square Med. School, Edinburgh – lectures are delivered twice a week by.... [?].

Natural Philosophy, since about six years, has also formed a part of the medical curriculum.

Those who make choice of the Med. profession, must not expect to repose on a bed of roses; they must be prepared to forego every selfish feeling and to encounter without shirking, severe bodily fatigue and keen mental anxiety. Their constitution should be good, their tempers obliging, yet firm. And they must be able to retain under the most trying circumstances, presence of mind. 'No act, except that of war, requires so much intrepidity, courage and promptness in fudging and in acting as that of physic,' Dr. Mackintosh's address.

November, 28th 1836 – Today I left my apartment in Sacksville Street, after a residence of about five months and raised my Ebenezer in Union Court, Old Broad Street with Mr William Eccles, with whom I have... [?] ... an association for the practice of Hernia.

Tuesday. Revd. a letter from Lady Wellesley[212], inviting me to call and see her at Hurlingham House near Fulham –

---

[211] A briefcase in the Christmas window of London department store in 1992 was priced at three hundred pounds or about $450.00.

[212] Lady Wellesley was the Marchioness Wellesley, the second wife of Richard Colley Wellesley, who was first Marquis Wellesley and oldest brother of the Duke of Wellington. She was an American, by the name of Marianne (or Mary Anne) Patterson. She was the widow of a wealthy shopkeeper, one of three sisters from Baltimore who eventually married English peers. They had been among the leading

took a cab and rode out there. It is about four miles from London fine old house built of brick situated among, and surrounded by, highly cultivated & ornamented grounds, surrounded by an iron paling. The entrance by a handsome iron gateway with neat Porter's lodge. I was ushered into her Ladyship's presence, by a member of liveried lacquers [lackeys], who one after the other announced my name. I first however, sent in my card and a message was brought that the Marquis [Marchioness] would be glad to see me. She received me with great cordiality and kindness shaking my hand with a regular English heartiness – I had a long conversation with her in which she evidenced for my success in a business and made many inquiries about it: and my reception by the faculty to whom she had given me letters. Says Sir Mm. Tierney[213] was delighted with me, that Mr Smith[214] of Richmond will send his cases of Hernia to me, that a nobleman of her acquaintance suffers under that disease, and that she will endeavour through his wife to get him to apply to me.

She than gave me a long account of her travels after health since I left her in Paris.

At Brussels she applied to a Dr, a homeopathist, who in the course of six weeks relieved her of complaints which the best medical men of England had failed to do. She took the 200th part of 1,000,000th of a grain Nuvomica – which produced no effect for 24 hours after that time for 60 hours great pain & stiffness of the muscles, then great relief of all her symptoms of disease. For an affection of the chest inflammation of the

---

admirers of and perhaps equally admired by the Duke of Wellington, himself. He was apparently most upset when Mrs. Patterson went to Ireland and married his older brother, the Lord Lieutenant of Ireland.

[213] Sir Matthew Tierney (1776-1845), a London physician who was admitted to the College of Physicians in 1806, was later appointed physician to the Prince of Wales and continued when he became George IV. He also was physician to King William IV.

[214] This may be Dr Thomas Southwood Smith (1788-1861).

bronchial vessels, she took an infinitesimal dose of Aconite, which had the same affect as a copious bleeding and in two days perfectly relieved her of the disease.

By following the plan of this Homeopathic she has regained, in a great measure, her health, she can eat more freely, digest better than before – is not subject to the violent & dreadful attacks of bilious Cholic to which she was formerly subject. Intestines, instead of constant and habitual constipation, producing intense headaches, which was only relieved by powerful purgations [?], act 'naturally, regularly, perfectly'. Facts are stubborn things.

Wednesday, November 30th, 1836 – I wrote to Camilla on Monday, stating that I should probably sail by the 16th Dec.

This morning recd. a letter from her and a P.S. by Mrs S. dated October 29th she has become a sage Femme – Sally a little vixion and makes her brother mind her.

Thursday, December lst, 1836 – Change of air or Pursuit of Health by Dr Jas. Johnson[215]. Etiolation or Blanching – Education – the present system of female education is a system of sensuality.

The Bourse of Paris, the rival of Neptune's Temple at Posidum, is one of the most noble of modern edifices. The moment it is entered, a noise resembling that of the distant roaring of the ocean in a storm is heard even when there are but few people moving about & conversing on the floor. This arises from its construction.

English trading vessels – the number, exclusive of the Royal Navy, 24,280 – the capacity of those vessels, 2,553,685 tons, and they give employment to 166,583 men and boys. In addition to the immense fleet just mentioned as actually

[215] Dr James Johnson wrote *Change of Air – Diary of a Philosopher 1831*, and in *The Economy of Health* in 1837 as well as many other articles.

belonging to British Ports, the British Empire possesses 333,579 ships of 214,878 tons, and 15,059 men, which belong to her colonies; so that, altogether the country possesses 27,859 merchant vessels.

Mr... dined with us today. He is a man who 'spent' some thirty years in buying and selling indigo and logwood. Having by this means accumulated an independence, he retired from business and since about ten years has devoted himself to the study of Latin & Greek, French and German languages to music and drawing to anatomy and Chemistry mechanics, geology, etc. He possesses industry but is exceedingly dull – and expresses himself with the greatest difficulty – loves to talk, thinks himself talented in no ordinary degree – as Lady W. says, "I was bored to extinction."

December 5th, 1836, Sunday – Went with Mr Eccles and Mr Myers, to Graves End[216] to see Mr. Davis. Started from London Bridge in the steam boat at ten in the morning, arrived about 12 1/2 o'clock, the distance by water is thirty miles down the river, by land it is about twenty. Graves End is situated on the river's edge in a low bottom, the ground rises as you recede from the water. Windmill Hill is a conical eminence, immediately behind and overlooking the town. I ascended the hill and had a beautiful view of town and river with its shipping – of country rich and cultivated and distant hills and woods. County of Kent. Dined with Davis at the Falcon Hotel and at four o'clock, took steamer for London and got home about 6 1/2. Went to Geo. Eccles and took supper.

The streets of Graves End are narrow & dirty, the houses small & ill built. It is a great place of resort for the Londoners in the summer season Particularly on Sunday!

---

[216] Gravesend was important as being the place where the customs' authorities recognised the port of London to begin; all ships, incoming and outgoing, were visited by officers there, and pilots embarked and disembarked at this port.

Friday last an old friend of Mr E. Came in from Gloucestershire – a plain blunt man a good specimen of an English Yeoman. He was dressed in a pair of drab small clothes & gaiters, buttoning up to his knee – thick shoes – quaker coat & long waistcoat etc. His thin strait hair hung over his collar behind and forehead in front; giving a rather pious look to his jolly and honest face. He had been a baker, but having acquired a property of about hundred a year, gave up business and now lives independently in the country; being (81) fond of hunting and a good shot, he is invited to the table of the neighbouring gentry & to their hunts. He speaks with a strong accent, and uses many provincialisms which are certainly unintelligible to me. In conversing with a French gentleman who was present, I had occasion to use the little of his language I knew. This excited the curiosity of Mr Best who in his peculiar language said, "Be'ast thou really a Yankee now? Why those speak as good English as I do, and better than thuch thou speaks the French – When didst thou learn to speak so many tongues!" When I told him that the Americans all spoke English he was exceedingly amazed.

There was another queer character came in Friday evening, named Mr Corvella, a fat pursy, ridiculous, old fellow. The very opposite of Shakespeare's Apothecary.

Monday, December 5th, 1836 – Revd. a letter from Mme C [his wife], anxious either to come to England or to have me come home – Dated November 4th Pottsville.

Visited Temple Lodge 19 – W. Eccles, W.M. Mr Weisbreich, S.

W. Vultuin – supper at 1… (?).

Wednesday, December 7th – Packed up my books and part of clothes etc. in black trunk, & put them on board a ship, S. Hannibel, Capt. G. Robert's care, sails from London, the 7th for New York. Called at Mr A. Stevenson's and left my passport for his signature.

Wrote to Lady Wellesley that I would do myself the honour of calling at Hurlingham H. on Friday to receive her command. Visited the Grand Lodge, Freemasons' Hall, Lord George Churchill M.W.D.G.M. A letter was read from the M.W.G.M. His Royal Highness the Duke of Sussex. etc.

9th – Went to see Lady W [ellesley].   M. Garct dined with us, and I promised to call & see his father who resides at Wisahickon, near Philad [elphia] – that is if convenient.

December 10, Saturday – left London in the steamboat Dart, at 6 a.m. for Boloryne[217], fair five shillings, obliged to put in to Ramsgate on account of the wind where we lay all night fine – harbour – full of ships masts – spent the evening on shore.

11th – Got into Boloryne about 10 a.m. and took my place in the Diligence for Paris at 1 p.m. where we arrived on Monday night at 11 1/2. Put up at the Hotel Windsor, Rue Rivoli.

12th – Dined with Dr. Herisson at the Café Anglais.
Took *dejeuner a la fourchette et a la Champagne.*

13th with him Dr. Nicker and Mr. Mancreve – got a new passport, the old one not having arrived from Boloryne bought two pair of boots and a hat – took my place for Le Havre at 5 p.m. When I arrived on the 14th at 4 p.m.
14th Wednesday.   Put up at the Hotel D'Amirante, where we stayed until the morning of the 19th.   When we got on board the good ship Charlemagne, Capt. Richardson bound for New York.

The above is the conclusion of Dr Carpenter's *1836 Diary of*

---

[217] Boulougne (sur Mer), on the coast of France.

London, except for the last page which contained the following receipt:

Beet Root – Nulle Plante Sarclie ne prepare mieux le sol pour les recoltes futures. On pent la cultiver dans presque tons les terrains; mais ceux qu elle prepare sont les solslegers, meubles, profonds, riches en humus tells que les terrains d'allervion.

La betterare blanche, *dite de* Silesie, *et la variete a* peau rose *et* a chair blanch, *sont les especes qui donnent le plus de just et le plus de sucre, et qui paraissent sons ton le rapports, meriter le preferance, pour la fabrication, et meme pour la niourriture des bestiaus.*